IT'S *NOT* ALL IN YOUR HEAD

Bruce and Eileen MacKenzie
with Linda Christie

IT'S *NOT* ALL IN YOUR HEAD

A Couple's Guide
to Overcoming Impotence

E. P. DUTTON NEW YORK

Although the authors and publisher have made every effort to ensure presentation of accurate and precise information, this book is not intended as an alternative to professional services, recommendations, or advice; neither does it imply an endorsement or recommendation of any or all of the alternative treatments and suggestions described.

The reader should first consult with a urologist specialist whose expertise includes experience with impotence with respect to any signs of chronic impotence and with a mental-health professional when diagnostically indicated.

Names, characters, places, dialogue, and events portrayed in this book are either the product of the authors' creation or are composites of certain conversations and events with names disguised to maintain anonymity.

IMPOTENTS ANONYMOUS (I.A.) and I-ANON are registered trademarks solely the property of Eileen and Bruce MacKenzie.

The Impotence Institute of America (I.I.A.) and the Impotence Institute International (I.I.I.) are "nonprofit, educational and charitable" organizations and are registered as 501-c-3 with the Internal Revenue Service. Both were incorporated in 1983.

Published in the United States by E. P. Dutton,
a division of NAL Penguin Inc.,
2 Park Avenue, New York, N.Y. 10016.

Published simultaneously in Canada
by Fitzhenry and Whiteside, Limited, Toronto.

Library of Congress Cataloging-in-Publication Data
MacKenzie, Bruce.
It's not all in your head.
1. Impotence—Popular works. 2. Impotence—Treatment.
I. MacKenzie, Eileen. II. Christie, Linda. III. Title.
RC560.I45M33 1988 616.6'92 87-24592
ISBN: 0-525-24649-5

Designed by REM studios

1 3 5 7 9 10 8 6 4 2

First Edition

This book is dedicated to—

the more than 10 million men in the United States of America and
their partners, together with the worldwide population, who suffer from chronic impotence in silence, secrecy, and shame
. . . needlessly!

CONTENTS

ACKNOWLEDGMENTS

To Myron I. Murdock, M.D., our very dear friend and urologist who gave us our first technical information concerning impotence and continues to educate us; contributes his time to serving as National Medical Advisor to Impotents Anonymous (I.A.) and I-Anon; became an incorporating officer of the Impotence Institute of America and the Impotence Institute International; agreed to write the book *Impotents Anonymous* and is the chief medical-information contributor and advisor to this book and wrote its foreword, our endless thanks for making possible our continuing contribution to the cause of combatting impotence.

For their editorial assistance we express appreciation and thanks to: Stephen M. Auerbach, M.D., Newport Beach, CA; Rose A. Axelrod, Silver Spring, MD; Mary Ann Bartusis, M.D., Langhorne, PA; Richard L. Fein, M.D., North Miami, FL; Matis A. Fermaglich, M.D., Teaneck, NJ; William P. Fitch III, M.D., San Antonio, TX; Irwin Goldstein, M.D., Boston, MA; R. Evan Jackson, Ph.D., Maryville, TN; Robert J. Krane, M.D., Boston, MA; William R. LaRosa, Jr., Clearwater, FL; James R. Leach, M.D., Tulsa, OK; Arnold Melman, M.D., New York, NY; Donald Motzkin, M.D., Van Nuys, CA; Uri P. Peles, M.D., Beverly Hills, CA; Maurice Sandler, M.D., San Pablo, CA; James K. Smolev, M.D., Baltimore, MD; Doug Stein, M.D., Tampa, FL; J. Douglas Trapp, M.D., Nashville, TN; E. Douglas Whitehead, M.D., New York, NY; and Adrian W. Zorgniotti, M.D., New York, NY.

We are truly grateful for the ongoing support and material supplied by the Associate Members of the Impotence Institute of America, Inc.: American Medical Systems, Astro-Lube, Inc., Bard Urological, Biosonics, Inc., Dacomed Corporation, E.K.C. Corporation, Gamogen, Inc., KSI Incorporated, Medical Engineering Corporation, Mentor Corporation, Osbon Medical Systems, Palisades Pharmaceutical Corporation, Repro-Med Systems, Inc., Revive Systems Corporation, Star Pharmaceuticals, Inc., and The Synergist Institute, Inc.

It has been estimated that 120,000 men received penile implants during the past five years (1983 through 1987), the same period in which Impotents Anonymous (I.A.) and I-Anon self-help chapters have existed. This compares with 50,000 men who received implants between 1960 and 1982. One explanation for this vast increase is the unprecedented media coverage given (and still being given) to I.A. and I-Anon, and their nonvested interest in impotence. We thank all the writers, directors, publishers, and technicians connected with newspapers, radio, television, and magazines (you know who you are) who contributed to the tremendous coverage.

Much of the content of this book—examples, explanations, and experiences—is the result of our exposure to, and communications with, the specially dedicated professionals and fellow impotent men and partners—a rapidly expanding "family." "Our story is their story." Because of anonymity we cannot individually thank the impotent men and their partners, but together we'll all continue to help other sufferers. Along with this "unidentified thanks" we express our appreciation to those very special Urologist Medical Advisors and Mental-Health Professionals who are taking that extra step in bringing the message to so many through the fellowship; and to Mark A. Immergut, M.D., the U.M.A. pioneer who has served the first I.A. and I-Anon chapters since January 1982.

FOREWORD

When people deal with impotence, the names of Eileen and Bruce MacKenzie quickly come to mind: in Australia on a television documentary; in Florida at a seminar; in Great Britain with the BBC; on two segments for the NBC "Today" show; and with more than seventy thousand impotent men and partners coming to grips with impotence.

In addition to filling roles as international spokespersons and authors, Eileen, as executive director of Impotents Anonymous (I.A.) and I-Anon, travels extensively opening new I.A. and I-Anon chapters. Bruce, as president of the institutes, works with membership, statistics, and development. They fulfill speaking engagements and participate in television, radio, magazine, and newspaper activities.

It's Not *All in Your Head* brings to the reader the most information ever presented from personal experiences with impotence. It has been gathered by the MacKenzies during their exposure to the thousands of impotent men, partners of impotent men, and those who have taken care of them (including mental-health professionals and over three thousand urological specialists).

Eileen and Bruce MacKenzie introduce the self-help, anonymous fellowship, patterned after successful applications in other fields, to impotence sufferers. They also make available total care for the treatment of impotence through the efforts of the institutes.

Eileen and Bruce continue to do much for many—the sufferers as well as those professionals, facilities, and manufacturers involved in the treatment of impotence.

Readers of this book will be sure to find examples and circumstances to which they can relate. *It's* Not *All in Your Head* is told by an impotent man and his partner who "walked in the shoes" of those who suffer, learned that "help *is* available," and overcame the effects of his chronic impotence. Eileen and Bruce MacKenzie continue to reach out to others with the message "Today, no man need remain chronically impotent!"

MYRON I. MURDOCK, M.D.

Director
IMPOTENCE INSTITUTE OF AMERICA, INC.

National Medical Advisor
IMPOTENTS ANONYMOUS (I.A.)
and I-ANON

IT'S *NOT* ALL IN YOUR HEAD

WHAT THIS BOOK WILL REVEAL TO YOU

Chronic impotence affects at least 10 million American couples. Living with this problem can shatter your self-esteem, undermine your relationships, and leave you angry, frustrated, and isolated from the world. We know—we went through it ourselves.

Millions of people are experiencing this same problem, not knowing where to turn or to whom to talk. Feeling alone, feeling their lives are falling apart, some turn to alcohol, and many divorce. An unfortunate few even commit suicide.

There is no need for a man to remain chronically impotent. No man need be incapable of maintaining an erection through the completion of successful intercourse. And his partner need not forfeit intimate sexual fulfillment. We want you to know that there *is* hope and there *is* help. You *can* find the right doctor, who will help restore your lives to normal.

Only a few years ago most couples with impotence problems had few options. But now you have many alternatives: medication, microsurgery, sex therapy, penile implants, external management, injection programs, and other technological developments.

You are not alone. Since we started Impotents Anonymous (I.A.) for men and I-Anon for wives and partners in 1982, we have received at headquarters (119 South Ruth Street, Maryville, TN 37801) more than sixty-thousand letters from men and women in the United States and from around the world. And every day we receive telephone calls from men and women in desperate need of accurate information and advice.

Reaching a successful resolution requires the active participation of both partners. Often we find that the partner seeks help before the impotent man. Using her own initiative, she may attend I-Anon meetings or read books to find out what help is available. Having taken the initial step, the partner often convinces the impotent man to come to an I.A. meeting or to consult with a urologist who specializes in impotence.

In this book we shall share what we, as a couple going through this life crisis, learned. And we shall share anonymously the concerns, fears, experiences, misconceptions, and success stories of hundreds of men and women we and our I.A. and I-Anon support groups have helped. We want to help you come to grips with your concerns, worries, and fears about you or your partner—fears that logic deems reasonable—but fears that in most cases are unfounded.

We shall explode the twelve common myths about impotence, including:

MYTH: It's all in your head.
FACT: More than half of all impotence (and some experts feel as much as 65 to 75 percent) results

from a physical problem that generally can be helped by medical treatment.

MYTH: Impotence can be overcome by taking a vacation or by having a few drinks to relax.
FACT: Impotence rarely responds to the common recommendation, "Just relax, you're trying too hard." Or: "You're under a lot of stress. You just need to get away for a while."

MYTH: Nothing can be done about impotence.
FACT: Almost without exception all impotent men can regain their ability to maintain an erection.

MYTH: You're getting older, what do you expect?
FACT: Some men under twenty are affected; others over eighty are not. The aging process, not age itself, may explain the onset of impotence.

It's Not *All in Your Head* explores all the new tests and treatments. We shall take you step by step through the entire process from finding the right doctor and support groups to understanding the causes for male impotence. You'll learn how to ensure a proper diagnosis. You'll learn—from impotent men and their partners—the pros and cons of various treatment methods. We'll even go beyond the medical resolution to help you readjust to your relationship as a couple, and to your life.

You'll find out, as we and hundreds of other men and women have done, how both of you can and should take an active part in planning a personalized treatment program that fits your medical, emotional, and financial needs.

We also want to share with you, anonymously, many letters we've received from men and women asking "What should I do?" Perhaps by reading their concerns and questions, and from hearing our advice and encouragement, you will learn better methods for coping with and resolving your problem.

Bruce has "walked in the impotent man's shoes." And Eileen has "walked in the partner's shoes." We have traveled overseas, in the United States, from coast to coast, north to south, meeting with professionals, opening I.A. and I-Anon chapters, speaking at professional seminars and meetings, and appearing on numerous radio and television talk shows. We have revealed our personal story and have talked about and shared—on national television and in magazine articles—almost every experience of the impotent man and his partner. And now we want to reveal to you what we've learned.

There is no reason for a man to remain chronically impotent. Successful lovemaking and sexual fulfillment are within your reach.

EILEEN V. MACKENZIE
Executive Director
IMPOTENTS ANONYMOUS (I.A.) and I-ANON
Maryville, Tennessee

BRUCE A. MACKENZIE
Founder and President
IMPOTENCE INSTITUTE OF AMERICA, INC.
and IMPOTENCE INSTITUTE
INTERNATIONAL, INC.
Maryville, Tennessee

HOW WE DISCOVERED THE SECRETS OF SUCCESSFUL TREATMENT FOR IMPOTENCE

EILEEN'S STORY

I began to grow skeptical of the accepted methods for treatment when after four years of sex therapy and my *tender loving care,* Bruce was still unable to consummate our marriage.

It was on our wedding night in 1977 that I first realized Bruce couldn't have an erection. But because Bruce had been recently widowed after twenty-four years of marriage to an alcoholic who died from the disease, I felt his problem was understandable. With the trauma of his loss and with three teenagers to rear, we both thought his impotence had been brought on by stress.

I felt that with tender loving care and with the restoration of a peaceful way of life, we could resolve the problem ourselves. Looking back on it, we *played doctor:* We *assumed* what caused Bruce's impotence, and we *assumed* what treatment was best.

After a year, Bruce had made no progress. He still could not gain or maintain an erection, and we still had not had successful intercourse. I was getting pretty uptight and angry. But I continued to play doctor: I believed Bruce's impotence was psychological. Fortunately Bruce and I could talk with one another about the problem, so eventually we decided to see our family physician.

Our doctor went right along with us. He too felt Bruce's problem was emotional, and indicated that physical problems are rare (a belief we later found to be *totally incorrect*). When the doctor's counseling efforts failed, I was even more depressed and angry. I was wondering, what's wrong with this man? And I felt cheated that Bruce hadn't told me about his problem *before* we got married. I was relieved when our doctor referred us to sex therapists. They should know what to do.

But nothing changed. After months of failure, Bruce was becoming even more difficult to live with, and I'm sure I was too. We would create arguments to prevent romantic involvement, we'd argue about anything. After a while I found the manual and oral techniques the sex therapists suggested as the sole means of lovemaking offensive. It wasn't the same kind of sharing a couple enjoys with sexual intercourse. I felt used, and I was fed up with doctors prying into my sexual desires—there wasn't anything wrong with *me!* I kept wondering why they didn't tell Bruce what to do; it was *his* fault, *not* mine. I was becoming more and more frustrated, and Bruce didn't seem all that interested in correcting his problem.

After nearly four years of not being able to consummate our marriage, after four years without the intimacy of lovemaking, and after spending a great deal of time and money on therapy, I had become detached and disinterested. I didn't want any more failures.

Finally the sex therapists suggested that we just *might* want to consult a urologist. Perhaps Bruce's diabetes could be causing a problem. Well, we jumped on it. Fortunately, and quite by chance, we consulted with a urologist who knew how to diagnose and treat impotence. (Less than one in three urologists specializes in the treatment of impotence.) The doctor found that Bruce's diabetes had caused irreversible nerve and blood-flow damage. No amount of sex therapy could have ever restored his potency!

When I heard the diagnosis, my first reaction was "Thank God, at least it's not in his head!" Then I had to deal with my anger. I felt cheated by the years of counseling before a urological evaluation was suggested. I also had to deal with my who-gives-a-damn attitude about sexual intimacy, which had built up over the years.

Fortunately, Bruce and I had learned through our Al-Anon experience how to be emotionally open and honest with one another; we could discuss our anger and resentment, work out our problems.

It was through our experiences that we realized the need for and the importance of starting Impotents Anonymous (I.A.) and I-Anon.

BRUCE'S STORY

When my condition worsened during the nine months preceding my wife's death, my *logic* told me that the turmoil of living with an alcoholic was affecting my sexual desire. Sometime later, though, I found myself in the embarrassing position of not being able to consummate my new marriage with Eileen.

When this happened, I made my *first mistake*: I exercised logic. I rationalized that my inability to maintain an erection was only natural—after all, I had lost my wife after twenty-four years of marriage; I had a horrible last few months with her dying from alcoholism; and I was left with three teenage children to rear. Both Eileen and

I agreed that some normal living and tender loving care should work wonders.

After a few months passed, though, I knew that things weren't right; that I was disappointing Eileen as well as myself. So I tried to compensate with more caressing and sexual foreplay. And I continued to reason that there couldn't be anything *physically* wrong with me, because I didn't have any symptoms other than the impotence.

After a year of repeated failure, I made my *second mistake,* though I didn't know it at the time. I got up enough nerve to go to my general practitioner. I now know that he didn't specialize in impotence. Even though he was aware of my diabetes—a major cause of impotence—he just assumed, as Eileen and I had, that I was among the 85 to 90 percent of men thought, in those days, to have psychogenic impotence; a popular but inaccurate belief. (Today, more and more evidence supports a far lower percentage.)

My *third mistake* was believing our general practitioner could provide counseling for this problem—more time and money spent without results.

My *fourth mistake* was taking his advice to get sex therapy without first being medically tested. From the fall of 1977 to the end of 1980 we tried one technique after another to lessen tension, to take away pressure. The sex therapists said, "You can't *will* an erection." They recommended joint masturbation and oral intercourse as a substitute for penile-vaginal intercourse. They told us, "If you get an erection, don't use it. Don't scare it away. If you get one, you'll get more. Later you can *use* the erection." In a strange sort of way, this advice encouraged my procrastination. The therapists reinforced the "logic" behind my idea that my problem was psychological.

As long as Eileen seemed happy, I didn't worry about it. As a man I could be sexually satisfied with sexual foreplay, orgasm, and ejaculation. What I didn't fully appreciate, but learned later, was that as a woman Eileen needed the joining and intimacy of lovemaking as much or more than the physical climax—fulfillment I could not give her.

We both became more and more crabby. Every time we had an argument, I got *my problem* thrown up in my face. I felt ashamed and at times became despondent. I started running everyone else's business—it was easier to run theirs than my own.

Finally the sex therapists suggested that "just perhaps" we might want to check with a urologist. They thought my diabetes could be playing a part. This was the very *first* time anyone suggested that my impotence might not be psychogenic!

By sheer luck, narrowly avoiding a *fifth mistake,* we went to a urologist who knew how to diagnose and treat impotence. After taking a medical history, conducting a thorough examination, and performing the appropriate tests, he declared I was physically impotent because of my diabetes. He gave me two choices: continue without penile-vaginal intercourse or opt for a penile implant. I knew nothing about the implant, but I knew I didn't like the first choice. So, after suffering through four years of false starts and dashed hopes, in the summer of 1981 I received my implant.

While I was in the hospital, I met two men who'd experienced virtually the same difficulties I'd had in finding accurate information, avoiding false starts, and obtaining valid help. I, like other men with this problem, felt isolated: To whom could I talk? To whom could I turn when I failed to get erections? Where could I get the truth?

I suddenly associated the similarities between the problems encountered by impotent men and their partners and those experienced by alcoholics and their partners. Both Eileen and I had learned to cope as partners with the illness of alcoholism through Al-Anon; that's where we first met. I asked myself, why couldn't a similar self-help fellowship work for impotent men and their partners? It was then that I conceived Impotents Anonymous (I.A.) and I-Anon, patterned after Alcoholics Anonymous (AA) and Al-Anon. I called Eileen from my hospital bed and said, "If you will start I-Anon, I will start Impotents Anonymous."

THE BIRTH OF IMPOTENTS ANONYMOUS (I.A.) AND I-ANON

"I can't talk about my impotence."
"I can't even discuss impotence with my best friend."
"I can't betray that my husband isn't making love to me."
"I can't admit I'm not macho anymore."
"I feel like a freak."

At an Impotents Anonymous meeting everyone can relax in the company of people who are experiencing the same problems. I.A. and I-Anon are self-help programs that give people an opportunity to talk to people "who have walked in the shoes of the person having the difficulty." I.A. and I-Anon give impotent men and their partners tremendous insight, compassion, and support, while preserving their dignity and anonymity.

In January 1982 our first chapter met at Suburban Hospital in Bethesda, Maryland. At that time, our sole objective was to prevent impotent men and their partners from wasting time and money. We encouraged them to seek an accurate diagnosis from a qualified urologist. When *The Washington Post* ran a syndicated story about our chapter's success, we started receiving inquiries for help and about starting similar programs around the country.

Almost before we knew it, we'd grown from one local effort to a nonprofit corporation with more than one hundred chapters nationwide.

OUR FIVE-POINT FORMULA FOR SUCCESSFUL TREATMENT

The secret to I.A. and I-Anon's success lies in the five-point formula for *your* success:

1. *Don't wait,* hoping that things will get better without professional treatment. Impotence is a symptom of a serious and sometimes life-threatening disease that requires professional treatment.
2. *Do not play doctor* by diagnosing yourself and prescribing your own treatment.
3. *Go directly to a urologist* specializing in the diagnosis and treatment of impotence problems.
4. *Act on the specialist's advice:*
   If you have a psychogenic problem, get counseling.
   If you have a physical problem, get medical treatment.
   If you have a physical problem and a psychological problem, get medical treatment and counseling.
5. *Remember, regaining your erection is only the beginning* of your recovery. You must also overcome the effects that impotence has had on your partner and on your life.

Follow this formula and you, like us and the thousands we've helped, will once again find sexual fulfillment.

As Bruce says, "I'm alive and well and doing a lot better than Mother Nature ever did for me."

And as Eileen says, "It's great to have a complete relationship again."

1

DISPELLING THE MYTHS OF IMPOTENCE

Today we estimate that physical problems account for 65 to 75 percent of chronic impotence. We also know that with proper diagnosis and treatment, most men can overcome the effects of impotence.

However, because being unable to have an erection is so embarrassing and because most people still believe that the problem is emotional, most men do not seek professional help. They choose instead to *stay in the closet* until the relationship with their partner deteriorates, or until they suffer so much personal humiliation and pain they can no longer cope.

Unfortunately, when men do muster enough courage to seek professional advice, they are often misinformed: "Just relax, you're trying too hard"; or, "You're getting older. What do you expect?" Thinking their situation is hopeless, they frequently drift back into the shadows.

In this chapter, we wish to dispel many of the common myths about chronic impotence. We find that when people know the truth about impotence, they can take positive action to correct their problem. And we find that the partners, relieved at learning they are not the cause of the problem, can respond more appropriately to their loved one's situation.

MYTH 1: IT'S ALL IN YOUR HEAD

Twenty years ago, absence of supporting medical evidence to the contrary resulted in the belief that 85 to 90 percent of impotence was psychologically based. However, current medical evidence supports estimates that perhaps more than 60 percent of chronically impotent men suffer from physical problems!

Unfortunately, though, most of us grew up believing that sexual problems are "in your head." So the majority of people experiencing impotence make the same mistake we did and assume that stress is taking a toll on their sex life. Most people experience enough stress in life that it's easy to rationalize a psychogenic cause.

Several clues, however, may alert you to the true nature of your impotence.

Signs of Psychogenic Impotence

If the onset of your impotence was sudden, perhaps after the death of a spouse or following another life crisis, then you may be experiencing *temporary* impotence. Your situation may resolve itself after a short recovery period or some counseling. If not, proper evaluation may indicate chronic psychogenic impotence.

If you can have sex with some partners and not with others, you are probably suffering from psychogenic impotence.

If you have erections during your sleep, you may have

psychogenic impotence. (This may be misleading, because your nighttime erections might last only thirty seconds or so rather than thirty to forty minutes, possibly indicating a physiological problem.)

If you can masturbate and maintain an erection through ejaculation, again you are probably psychogenically impotent.

Signs of Organic Impotence

If your sexual performance gradually deteriorated with time, your impotence most likely has an organic source.

If you are not having erections during your sleep, there may be an organic cause. Normally men have from three to five erections, each lasting thirty to forty minutes during dream (REM, or rapid eye movement) sleep.

If you cannot masturbate and maintain an erection through ejaculation, then you probably have an organic problem.

Regardless of your history and symptoms, if you remain impotent for more than five or six weeks, you should suspect chronic impotence and seek a medical evaluation from a urologist who specializes in impotence. You cannot expect chronic organic impotence to reverse itself with time. More about that later.

MYTH 2: IMPOTENCE CAN BE OVERCOME BY TAKING A VACATION OR BY HAVING A FEW DRINKS TO RELAX

If you suffer from temporary (situational) impotence caused by excess stress or fatigue, taking a vacation might help you relax and increase your sexual desire. If you are chronically impotent, however, this "prescription" will not help. Going away for a few weeks isn't going to change things that much.

If a couple of drinks would help an impotent man, everyone would have two drinks! Like a vacation, alcohol may help you relax after a stressful day and increase your sexual interest. However, because alcohol is a depressant, it may further impair your performance. Every partner of an alcoholic knows "the promise received at the bottom of the stairs" and "the failure at the top of the stairs."

If your impotence persists for five weeks or more, don't play doctor. Seek a professional evaluation.

MYTH 3: IT'S ALL MY PARTNER'S FAULT

Impotence often creates emotional problems that affect the relationship. Often the man will rationalize his impotence by saying, "Gee, this is old hat. I need something new and intriguing . . . a surprise." Or he may become supercritical, saying "My wife is too fat," or, "My wife is too skinny. She doesn't turn me on anymore."

The impotent man may firmly believe that if he had another partner, things would be different. Something inside his head, though, usually tells him not to put it to the test: "Don't try it, buddy. You are going to fail there also." If that happens, his last excuse will be blown out of the water. He doesn't want any more failures.

In response to the man's criticism, the partner often accepts responsibility for causing the problem. The harder she tries to placate him, however, the more he resorts to manipulation and control. When the partner accepts responsibility for causing the impotence problem, often the man does not feel compelled to look at himself and does not admit he has an impotence problem. In effect, the partner actually is helping him procrastinate.

The result is a downward spiral.

MYTH 4: IF HE LOVED ME, HE WOULD MAKE LOVE TO ME

We get many calls from heartbroken partners: "I think I could survive without sexual intercourse, if only he would tell me he loves me. If he'd just put his arm around me, or tell me that I'm pretty . . . just give me a little sign that he cares."

These women are shocked when we tell them that his behavior is quite natural. Think for a minute. He comes home, sees you in a pretty dress, and gives you a compliment. You smile and give him a hug, a peck on the cheek. Before you know it, you are engaging in sensual activities that lead you to the bedroom *and* to another failure. Although he may love you very dearly, he will find that it's *safer* to treat you as a sister or even a brother.

Many partners start to believe: *If he has sex with me, it proves that he loves me;* or the converse: *If he does not have sex with me, it proves that he does not love me, or that his affections are going elsewhere.* The partner begins to believe "I'm unable to attract him or turn him on." She starts carrying the burden of guilt: "What am I doing wrong?" She may even begin to wonder if she can still turn on a man.

We find that, unlike partners with impotence problems, the majority of "normal" people in loving relationships do not equate love with the sexual act. In fact, even in bad relationships partners may continue to have sex *without* love. Love and sex tend to reinforce one another; however, *having sex does not prove your love.*

MYTH 5: VITAMINS WILL MAKE ME POTENT

Every time you turn on the television, you see messages telling you to eat more fiber, drink more milk, get plenty of vitamins and exercise, and so forth. When you begin to have erection failures, it's only natural for you to think

"Maybe I'm lacking something." Because many people have been led to believe that vitamins can do miracles, they play doctor and prescribe vitamins to solve the problem. Sometimes doctors even reinforce this decision by saying "Go ahead. Vitamins won't do any harm."

There is no evidence, however, that vitamins improve erectile function. Don't play doctor, get a medical evaluation.

MYTH 6: MASTURBATION CAUSES IMPOTENCE

Unfortunately, many of us, as children, were told that masturbation is sinful; that terrible things would happen to us if we indulged in these "selfish" and "sinful" pleasures. You may not recall this for years; but when you become impotent, you may think, "Oh, God, I was told it was sinful. Now I'm being punished." This is just a fallacy fostered by old wives' tales. Masturbation does not cause impotence. The saying "Use it or lose it" is also false. Impotence is not caused by a lack of sexual activity.

MYTH 7: IMPOTENCE WILL GO AWAY WITH TIME

We believe the myth that impotence will go away with time persists primarily because, in the past, medical schools did not educate doctors about impotence. Because most doctors were taught that impotence is almost always psychogenic, they don't want to become involved with it. So doctors have virtually ignored, evaded, and not talked about impotence. It's often easier for doctors to say "It took a while coming on, so it will take a while to go away."

To the contrary, we find that waiting may cause more problems. For example, you may experience a few erection failures and begin to worry about what's going to happen the next time. Your fear of failure may then become a self-fulfilling prophecy that creates your next failure. Soon this growing psychogenic overlay creates an even worse problem.

In a few cases where stress or tension results in temporary impotence, letting time pass and allowing the stress to subside may resolve the problem. However, this applies to a very small percentage of men. Be awfully careful before you fritter away valuable time. Check it out.

MYTH 8: AGE CAUSES IMPOTENCE

Some men in their nineties do very well and some men in their twenties are impotent. When we hear that a doctor has told someone, *You're getting older. You're just slowing down,* we ask them, "Did you ask your doctor, *Gee, has it happened to you?*" Age in itself is not a factor in impotence. The effects of the *aging process,* however, may be a factor: hardening of the arteries, neuropathy (see Glossary, pp. 175–181, for definitions of medical terms), and so forth—but not to everybody. Also, we are not aware of any direct correlation between the so-called male menopause and impotence. Don't assume or accept that impotence is an inevitable and natural result of growing older.

MYTH 9: TAKING HORMONES WILL CURE IMPOTENCE

Many impotent men really believe that their hormonal level must be low, so taking hormones will restore their erection ability. Taking hormones, usually testosterone, is helpful for the 3 or 4 percent of men with diagnosed hormonal deficiencies. This is, however, a *very small percentage* of cases. Later in this book we'll discuss the various tests used to diagnose hormonal problems.

MYTH 10: TENDER LOVING CARE WILL OVERCOME IMPOTENCE

Eileen can personally vouch that TLC will not overcome impotence. In those cases where the man is experiencing a temporary loss of desire due to depression, anxiety, and so forth, TLC may help him through this period. And TLC will help the chronically impotent man retain his self-esteem and self-worth.

Impotents Anonymous and I-Anon meetings offer TLC to men and their partners: You learn a lot of facts, you become comfortable using the word *impotence,* you find out that you are not a freak, and you learn that treatment is available. But even this TLC will not cure your chronic impotence.

TLC may also have a downside, misleading the man into thinking that his partner is perfectly satisfied with things the way they are. Her kindness and love may make him think she's not concerned about it, so he doesn't have to do anything about it. But when she sees that her TLC is not producing positive results, her kindness gradually will decline. Eileen tells I-Anon groups that she finally gave up on TLC: "What good did it do anyway?"

We have to keep in mind that couples respond to impotence in a number of ways. Some couples adjust to impotence by becoming companions and friends; there isn't a great desire to overcome the impotence. Some couples just roll with the punches and learn to enjoy sex without penile-vaginal intimacy. But the majority of the men and women we've talked to indicate they would like to continue with the penile-vaginal sexual relationship they had earlier enjoyed.

MYTH 11: OVERCOMING IMPOTENCE WILL FIX EVERYTHING WRONG WITH MY LIFE

Resolving your impotence only restores your ability to have intercourse. All of the emotional problems that have developed during the years of an unsatisfactory relationship will not go away overnight. Your partner isn't going to sit back and say, "Oh, now everything is great."

Involving the partner in the medical diagnosis and treatment decisions helps prepare her for change, especially if the man decides to get a penile implant. Although penile implants are totally concealed, Eileen was "grossed out" the first time she "saw" an implant: "The doctor had me operate Bruce's implant after his surgery. If I'd had some preparation, the shock would not have been nearly so traumatic."

I.A. and I-Anon meetings are especially helpful to couples going through this period of transition and adjustment. A support group can answer those personal questions you choose not to ask your doctor. Besides, while doctors may have professional expertise, they haven't "walked in the shoes of the impotent man" or in those of the partner.

Many people need *psychological counseling* to help them deal with the psychogenic overlays of impotence. One couple who comes to mind drove over five hours to attend each I.A. meeting. The man was very demanding, banging on the table to stress every point. As they continued to come, though, he heard other people saying what his wife said. He began to realize that what she said had the "ring of truth." His wife finally realized that she too had legitimate needs. One night she told him to "shut up." He was thunderstruck.

We recommended they get marriage counseling before pursuing treatment for his impotence. Several months later she called, saying "I can't thank you enough.

Our situation has changed so much. Life is becoming so peaceful, we can talk now. And we're going to a urologist next week for an evaluation."

Overcoming the effects of impotence is only the first step in starting your new relationship.

MYTH 12: NOTHING CAN BE DONE ABOUT IMPOTENCE

The myth that nothing can be done about impotence is totally wrong! "Well, nothing can be done about it. There are other things in life to enjoy" is usually heard from professionals who don't treat impotence; or from well-meaning friends who simply don't know what they are talking about.

If *you* believe it's hopeless, it's a cop-out! You really do not want to do anything about your impotence problem.

Thanks to medical advances, it's no longer a question of *can I or can't I* but *will I or won't I get help.* Generally speaking, *there is no reason for anyone to remain chronically impotent.*

The following chapters will show you step by step how to build the groundwork for a successful treatment plan. We will tell you how to:

Get the best diagnosis and treatment available.
Participate in your diagnosis and treatment decisions.
Handle your life, your impotence, *and* your relationship.
Realize the sexual fulfillment you and your partner deserve.

So now let's begin to identify the key steps toward *your* personalized treatment plan.

2

WHAT'S HAPPENING TO US?

"I believe I could get by without having intercourse," Kate said. "But what drives me up the wall is that Brian no longer tells me he loves me."

"My husband won't even put his arm around me," Helen added.

Stefanie chimed in, "Last week I bought the cutest dress to wear to our class reunion, and he didn't even notice." She turned to Eileen MacKenzie, seated at the head of the table, and asked, "Did you and Bruce go through this?"

"We sure did," Eileen assured the I-Anon group. "And more. At night around bedtime, I made sure we started arguing about something. If we went to bed angry, we wouldn't make love, and we wouldn't have to face another failure. Finally I even convinced myself that I didn't care about having sex any more. I told myself that I had more important things to do at my age."

"I can relate to that," Stefanie said. "But why do men act this way?"

"They have to," Eileen said. "Consider the situation. If your husband gives you a kiss, and tells you that he loves you, you respond and expect more endearments. He becomes fearful of another failure. He does not want the humiliation of leaving you frustrated. He cannot put himself in a position of incompetence in making love to you. Better he remain distant and not start something he cannot finish."

Impotence is not a condition that affects only the man. It affects the relationship. As the problem continues, the partner may become fearful and think perhaps her mate has grown indifferent to the relationship. Efforts to encourage lovemaking, or to discuss the problem, are of no avail and may lead her to take on the complete responsibility for her partner's impotence. Blaming herself, coupled with her growing feelings of guilt and anger, creates greater stress and helplessness.

Dyan, a woman we spoke with at an I.A. meeting, told us that she became so angry that she convinced her husband to switch partners with another couple. When he didn't want to, she became terrifically guilty about the incident. Only after they talked about this problem at an I.A. meeting were they able to deal with their true emotions. Another woman, Marcie, related at an I-Anon meeting that she became very insecure about her marriage when her husband, a busy attorney, moved out of their bedroom because "he needed a private place to work at night." Marcie was afraid to discuss his impotence, let alone to assert her own rights. Only after she obtained professional counseling could she understand the problem and begin to communicate with him.

On the other hand, Rachael, who called us at I.A. headquarters, said she felt terribly threatened when her paraplegic partner vowed to do something about his impotence. She was afraid that she would lose control over him, that he might seek another partner, once he regained his sexual ability. Later she called to report that their sex life was better than ever since he got his implant. After they received some counseling, she found that all her worries were for nothing.

COMMON REACTIONS TO IMPOTENCE

At some time in his life every man will experience temporary (situational) impotence. This is normal. He may be recovering from the flu, experiencing excessive stress at the office, or suffering from fatigue. Excessive drinking, worries, and marital discord can all take their toll. However, if the problem lasts five or more weeks, the couple should consider the real possibility that the condition is chronic. At that point, it's time to get an accurate diagnosis from a urologist who specializes in impotence.

Couples who wait, who spend many months and years struggling with chronic impotence, often find that their relationship begins to deteriorate under the strain. If you take prompt action, you will avoid many of the complications caused by the psychological overlays of impotence.

Avoiding Romantic Encounters

At first, the man and then eventually the woman will begin to avoid romantic encounters, to avoid experiencing another failure. Each failure is a painful reminder to the man of his thought that he isn't a complete man, that he's a "freak." And a painful reminder to the partner that possibly he doesn't care, that he may be having an affair with another woman, or that perhaps she has failed to remain attractive enough to arouse his lovemaking. He avoids taking her to candlelight dinners, telling her that she's pretty, putting his arm around her. They may, as we did, start little arguments before bedtime to squelch any romantic feelings and circumvent subsequent overtures.

At first the partner makes excuses: "Tony must be having problems at work." Or, "Jack's under a lot of stress." She may even attempt to draw her man into a discussion about it. But he'll often cut her off by saying "I'm not having any problems." This is extremely hurtful to the partner. Thinking she's done something wrong, she often will attempt to change the situation. Or she may feel guilty that after having such a good relationship for such a long time, she shouldn't be making such a fuss. But *women do feel rejected.*

Blaming Every Problem on the Lack of Good Sex

Brenda, an I-Anon member, explained it this way:

"If things are all right in the bedroom, they will be all right in the kitchen.

"If things are all right in the kitchen, they will be all right in the bedroom."

It's only natural for a couple experiencing an impotence problem to blame all kinds of troubles on the poor performance in the bedroom. How many times we've heard, "If you were a good lover . . ." After awhile, they begin to believe that if *the problem* were fixed, all of their other troubles would go away too.

As Craig said at an I.A. meeting, "After we overcame my impotence problem, we found out that everything does not pivot around the bedroom." It's true that understanding and overcoming your impotence problem will relieve a great deal of stress. Fixing Craig's penis, however, didn't automatically turn his life into a bed of roses. That took time and a little work on both their parts. It was worth it though.

Withdrawal from Family and Friends

Many times the man and even the partner begin to withdraw from their family and friends. "Living the lie" becomes too stressful.

As Eileen explained to an I-Anon group one evening, "I remember after Bruce and I were married, our friends and family would ask about us. I'd smile and say 'things are going great!' All the while, we both knew that things weren't going great, in the bedroom. Pretty soon I didn't want to be around these people. I didn't want to lie to them anymore."

Too often the man withdraws from his friends because he feels as if he's only half a man. As his self-esteem and self-worth dwindle, he may begin to dress shabbily, go unshaven, and shy away from social activities. Or sometimes the reverse happens, as in the case of a middle-aged manager, George, who became obsessed with his work and never had time for leisure.

George's wife, Aleen, built up a wall so she wouldn't be hurt. She started hobbies, did more things with the children, occupied the rest of her time with a career, and avoided being with her chronically impotent partner. This activity helped block out her anger and hurt.

Once you deal with your impotence problem, you will once again be able to return to the social life you yearn for.

THE FIVE STAGES OF IMPOTENCE

We find that couples experiencing impotence problems typically progress through five stages. The first stage includes denial, rationalization, and hope. When a couple is in this stage, we hear statements such as "I'm not impotent; I just can't have an erection." The second stage is characterized by depression, anger, and fear: "Why me?

What have I done to deserve this?" When the couple enters the third stage, they go through a period of searching and learning. They read books, talk to their doctor, and attend I.A. and I-Anon meetings. During the fourth stage they begin to reorganize their thinking about the problem. And during the fifth stage they decide what action to take about their problem.

When couples become stuck in one of these stages, they usually do not resolve their impotence problem. Unfortunately, when this happens, they either continue with a miserable existence or dissolve the relationship. Today there is every reason for achieving a happy ending. *No man* need remain chronically impotent, and more and more couples are finding this out. *Help is available.*

Stage 1: Denial, Rationalization, and Hope

If you are still in stage 1, you are not really convinced that you have an impotence problem. We hear many men say, "It only happens sometimes. What I need is a change. It will come back." Or, "It's my partner's fault. What I need is a pursuit (that is, the chase is more interesting than the capture); a woman who will excite me."

The man reasons that he didn't *injure* his penis, so it's only logical that it will begin working again under the "right" circumstances. Maybe he's having a tough time at work, the children are having problems, or he's out of work. "Who can make love with this going on?" he will think, or, "It's normal not to have romantic feelings under these circumstances." Many times we hear men say, "When things get better, things will return to normal."

In the meantime, the partner may be bringing added stress to herself in her efforts to ease his difficulties. For example, if money is a problem, she takes on extra work. Or she tries to make his homelife extra special by getting a new hairdo or fixing a candlelight dinner. Then they begin to avoid intimate situations. When her tender loving care doesn't seem to help, she may become disappointed or angry.

Stage 2: Depression, Anger, and Fear

If you are in stage 2, you are scared and angry.

Men begin to wonder, "Where am I going? What's happening to me? I'm a freak, one of a kind. I'm not a man *or* a woman—I'm an *it.*"

Younger men may even contemplate suicide. We've seen strong men break down and cry during this stage of their impotence.

This man begins to rebel against the whole world. He criticizes everyone and everything, especially his partner. Meg, who called I.A. for advice, said, "Michael just criticizes me all of the time. I can't do anything right." Men like Michael have a short fuse, a chip on their shoulder.

Though men in this stage are desperately afraid, they try not to worry about it. They rationalize that "It's just temporary." Their worst fear, however, is that it's *not* temporary. And they reason that "If it is not temporary, *it is forever.*"

Reacting to the man's withdrawal and depression, his partner may try to jolly him up. She usually does not attribute his depression to impotence, so she will dress well, try to look attractive, and so forth. When he doesn't respond, she doesn't understand why he is no longer affectionate. She may become depressed as Kathy did and say, "I've done all I can do; what more is there?" Or, "How much longer can I go on living this way?"

This is a very difficult time for the partner. She is afraid that she is becoming unattractive, that she's lost her sex appeal. Maybe she's taken her loving man for granted, and now he's bored or has found another woman. After secretly attending several I-Anon meetings, Leslie built up enough courage to talk to her husband about her fear that he had found someone else. She told him that because she was so depressed she had secretly been attending the I-Anon meetings. And she told him that she still loved him. At the next meeting, Leslie reported that her husband said he had been afraid to discuss it with her, and that it was a load off his shoulders to talk with her about it. Leslie said, "I don't mind so much that he is impotent, now that I know he loves me."

As Amanda, who had become angry, said at an I-Anon meeting: "I've given him the best years of my life, I've raised his children, I've worked to help buy our house, and now he's tossing me aside."

Like many partners, Amanda felt "used and abused," especially when her husband, Warren, appeared to be satisfied with oral sex and masturbation. For many women, sex *other* than penile-vaginal intercourse is no longer a sharing experience. She is not content with this form of lovemaking on a permanent basis, to the *exclusion* of intercourse. "He's getting his jollies" while she is not experiencing the closeness and the togetherness that intercourse provides.

These emotions don't come all at once. They build gradually over many months and lead to depression. Her anger and depression also affect her partner, and they end up caught in a vicious cycle.

Couples also feel isolated. You don't know to whom to talk. A man won't talk about it to his friends at the office or in the locker room. And the partner won't betray her husband, whom people think is perfectly normal. *Not to a single soul.* Besides, there is always a chance that his impotence is a reflection on her abilities as a wife. When the couple can't discuss the problem with each other, you have a double dose of isolation. Sharing your emotional fears can help. It certainly helped us through difficult times. At least we had each other.

Stage 3: Searching and Learning

Fortunately, more and more couples are reaching stage 3. Unfortunately, the advice they receive is often poor. Many try to play doctor by buying pills through a mail-order house or by taking vitamins. When these methods don't work, they often crawl back into their isolation, convinced that nothing can be done.

Today more and more people are getting very good advice. Physicians and mental-health professionals are becoming aware that *65 to 75 percent of impotence may involve a physical condition.* So, before wasting months and years waiting for the condition to reverse on its own or respond to sex therapy, doctors and therapists are referring people for a urological evaluation. Some people are getting good advice from I.A. and I-Anon meetings. And some are directly consulting a urologist who specializes in impotence. We hear more and more psychiatrists saying "Don't assume that it is in your head until your urologist tells you that it is."

It's vital that you do not try to play doctor. Go to a urologist who specializes in impotence to determine:

if you have a physical or psychogenic problem,
if the condition is reversible, and
what treatments are available.

If your relationship is in jeopardy or if your condition is psychogenic, get a referral to a marital counselor.

The searching and learning stage is an important one. It should not, however, become a tool for procrastination. At some point you need to leave the "twilight zone" where you fantasize the miraculous, spontaneous restoration of your potency. You need to introduce some humility, accept that you have a problem, and take positive action to overcome the effects of your impotence.

Stage 4: Reorganizing Your Thinking

Accepting that you have a chronic impotence problem does not mean that you are resigned to suffer with it. Nor does it mean that you intend to resolve the problem. Stage 4, *acceptance,* simply means that you recognize that due to either a medically diagnosed physical problem or a psychological problem, you are unable to achieve and maintain sufficient penile rigidity to penetrate and complete intercourse to the satisfaction of both partners.

Stage 5: Making Your Decision

Once you have truly accepted that you are chronically impotent, you have reached stage 5 and can make a decision about what you want to do about it.

You can choose to remain chronically impotent; or
if your condition is reversible, you can choose to undergo corrective treatment; or
if your condition is not reversible, you can choose to overcome the effects of your impotence.

Choosing a course of action is the man's decision. He must, however, be prepared to accept the effects of his choice on his partner because, in the light of his decision, she has the right to choose what future she wants for herself and for the relationship. Some couples report that they are able to have a satisfactory sex life without penile-vaginal intercourse. Limiting your sexual options in this way, however, is no longer necessary. *You do have a choice.*

IS IT FOREVER?

Almost without exception, every chronically impotent man can overcome the effects of impotence. For some men this will happen through the medical treatment of an injury or disease: controlling diabetes, restoring hormonal balance, or repairing damaged blood vessels. Others will gain satisfaction through the use of medication or aids such as injection therapy, external management devices, or penile implants. Many alternatives exist today. Every couple should be able to find the solution that best meets their physical and emotional needs.

In the next chapter, we shall tell you more about how to find the professional help you need to diagnose the nature of your problem and to help you overcome the effects of impotence.

3

FINDING THE RIGHT DOCTOR

Finding the *right* doctor is an important step toward getting a satisfactory diagnosis. We find, however, that *deciding* to find the right doctor is the *first* problem most couples must overcome.

WHEN SHOULD YOU BECOME CONCERNED ABOUT AN ERECTION PROBLEM?

"I'm not really sure that I am impotent," a man calling from southern California told Bruce on the telephone. "I'd really be embarrassed if I went to my doctor and he told me that I was worried about nothing."

This is a concern we hear from many men who are experiencing erection problems. Perhaps they don't have a problem every time they make love. Perhaps their penis enlarges (swells up) but doesn't become rigid enough to achieve penetration. Or perhaps their erection lasts for five minutes or so and then begins to lose stiffness. If any of these symptoms persist for five weeks or more, though, you may have a chronic impotence problem.

Impotence can be a side effect of a medical condition that may be very serious, even life-threatening. You wouldn't hesitate to see a doctor if you had a persistent sore throat or chronic cough. These "side effects" also can be symptoms of conditions needing medical attention. So why would you put off seeing the doctor about a problem with erections? Probably because of the lingering myth that "It's all in your head."

Well, it is *not* all in your head. So, to protect your health, you need to stop playing doctor and go to a qualified urologist for an accurate diagnosis.

FINDING A QUALIFIED PHYSICIAN

Many people consult with their family physician first. We did. He was the person we trusted; and though he was good, what he knew about impotence you could put in a thimble. As a result, we did not get proper help for nearly four years.

Others, believing there's a problem with their relationship, may seek psychological or marriage counseling first. Often the couple, as well as the therapist, assumes that the stresses associated with their life-style and with his impotence are impairing their relationship and aggravating the impotence problem. Their logic tells them that as he didn't injure his penis or hasn't been ill, stress must be the answer. These people are playing doctor.

Only one in three urologists in the United States specializes in impotence. Only these specialists have the knowledge, skill, and instruments necessary for making an accurate diagnosis. Fortunately, and quite by luck, Bruce went to a urologist specializing in impotence and received the help he needed.

You too can find a urologist specialist. We suggest that you consult with one or more of the following people and organizations to help you with your quest.

Your family physician. If you are more comfortable, see your family physician first for a complete physical. He or she can make certain that all of your organs and systems are working correctly. If, however, your family doctor does not pinpoint the cause of your impotence or correct the problem in a relatively short period of time, ask for a referral to a urologist who specializes in impotence.

Your local county medical society. Local medical organizations may maintain lists of urologists who are interested in impotence.

Impotence clinics. Impotence clinics can be extremely helpful. Most are staffed by professionals specializing in a variety of fields including urology, endocrinology, internal medicine, neurology, marriage counseling, sex therapy, and so forth. These professionals can accurately diagnose your problem and recommend a comprehensive medical and mental-health treatment program.

Clinics affiliated with hospitals and universities. Hospital and university clinics offer comprehensive programs similar to impotence clinics. While they may offer the best of all worlds for diagnosis and treatment, they may be expensive and time-consuming. In addition, you may need to travel some distance to find these clinics. Note, however, that some people actually prefer to seek help in distant communities because they feel doing so will better protect their anonymity.

Impotence device manufacturers. Sometimes people write or call device or pharmaceutical manufacturers for information or a physician referral. Many manufacturers offer informative brochures and physician referrals. If you do this, remember that manufacturers are in the business of selling their products, not in providing unbiased information about help for impotence.

Impotents Anonymous, I-Anon, Impotence Institute of America, and Impotence Institute International. The Impotence Institute of America and Impotence Institute International maintain lists of qualified urologist specialists and mental-health professionals. You can write to I.A., or I-Anon, or the institutes for a referral to a professional in or near your community.

Each month I.A. answers thousands of requests for information. In addition, the institutes publish pamphlets and a newsletter containing information about the diagnosis and treatment of impotence. The newsletter supplies information on the newest research and trends in the field.

There are more than one hundred local I.A. and I-Anon chapters located around the country. In addition to the members who have gone through what you have, each chapter has a lay coordinator and Urologist Medical Advisor who are available to listen and to address your questions and concerns at chapter meetings.

So help *is* available. It is up to you to reach out for it.

OUR TEN POOR-TREATMENT DANGER SIGNS

Many of you already may have received a diagnosis and course of treatment from a physician and/or mental-health professional. Or perhaps you are still going through the process and are having some doubts about whether you are receiving the best help available. The following ten poor-treatment danger signs may alert you to potential problems with your diagnosis and treatment:

1. *Does your physician offer both diagnostic and treatment services?* Some physicians do only diagnostic tests and never offer any treatment. We remember one man who

spent over $3,000 for tests only to find out that the doctor did not offer treatment. When you are selecting a doctor, make certain that if your problem is medical, the doctor will also treat your impotence.

2. *Is your diagnosis taking too long?* The medical diagnosis should take no longer than two months to complete. Most tests can be performed in the doctor's office. The physician should follow a logical order for performing the diagnostic tests. You should not receive every test in the book unless there is a reason for performing each of them (see Chapter 4 for more details). The physician also may refer you to a mental-health professional for a psychological evaluation. Once your physician makes his or her diagnosis, you should know whether your problem is physically or psychologically based.
3. *Were you examined and evaluated by a physician?* If your diagnosis is being handled by a paraprofessional (nurse, medical assistant, or person not having a medical degree), go to a different clinic. Only a urologist specialist can order appropriate tests and interpret their results.
4. *Was your medical treatment delivered by a qualified professional?* You should be treated by a licensed medical practitioner (M.D.). You should not be getting treatment from a pharmacist or from some company advertising potions, elixirs, aphrodisiacs, or devices in the back of a magazine. Or from someone selling black-market injections in a dark alley. Only a medical professional is qualified to treat your impotence problem. We recommend an A.U.A. board-certified urologist.
5. *Did your physician offer more than one treatment alternative?* If you have a physical problem, the urologist specialist should offer you a number of treatment alternatives and explain the pros and cons of each treatment plan *relative to your particular condition.* If the physician offers

only one treatment option—for example, one type of penile implant—you should ask for other options, or seek a second opinion. Later chapters will explain the many options available today.

If you have psychogenic impotence, the medical specialist should refer you to a qualified mental-health professional. A number of people with physical impotence can also benefit from counseling because of the psychogenic overlays that affect almost every couple having this problem.

6. *Has the physician involved your partner in the process?* At some point, a good doctor will include the partner in the process, at least to give information about the diagnosis and treatment options. She has the right to ask questions, to understand what is going on, and to know what to expect.
7. *Is your treatment taking too long?* Prolonged testosterone therapy is probably the most common complaint we hear from men. We received a call from one man whose doctor had been giving him testosterone injections for three years—*without any improvement in his condition.* If testosterone, the male sex hormone, does not work in two to three months, it probably never will work. Testosterone is helpful only for those men who have a diagnosed testosterone deficiency. This accounts for only 3 to 5 percent of impotent men. Taking testosterone when no deficiency is present will not improve *libido* (sex drive) or restore potency. Not only that, but long-term testosterone therapy poses some potentially serious side effects. More about testosterone therapy in a later chapter.
8. *Are you receiving psychological counseling, marriage counseling, or sex therapy without first having received a urological evaluation?* Because 65 to 75 percent of impotence stems from a physical problem, it is a mistake to get counseling before undergoing a complete medical evaluation.

We made this mistake and, as a consequence, we spent several frustrating, and expensive, years with no success. Remember, impotence *may be* a symptom of a potentially life-threatening disease process. You should always look for an underlying medical cause before you seek counseling.

9. *Is it difficult for you to discuss your problem with your doctor?* If you forget to ask your doctor questions during your appointment, call back. Or write down your questions to take to your next appointment. If your doctor is uncomfortable about talking with you and your partner, or if your doctor doesn't want to take the time to talk with you, find another doctor.
10. *Are you progressing at a satisfactory rate?* If you believe your diagnosis or treatment is taking too long, get another professional opinion. Attend an I.A. or I-Anon meeting, talk to others who've experienced what you have, or seek a second medical evaluation. Don't waste precious months and years as we did.

In the next chapter you will learn more about the diagnostic procedures your physician will use to determine if you have physical or psychogenic impotence. The more you know about these procedures, the better you will be able to help your physician understand your problem, and the better equipped you will be to understand the results of the evaluation.

4

EVALUATING IMPOTENCE

Impotence is not a disease; neither is it a primary ailment. Impotence may be a symptom of a serious disease process—diabetes, for example. Knowing how the penis gains and maintains an erection will help you understand how an injury or disease can disrupt this process. And it will help you understand the nature of the tests the urologist who specializes in impotence will perform to diagnose the cause of your impotence.

THE FORMULA FOR POTENCY

An erection begins when the brain sends signals to the blood vessels supplying the penis. These signals tell the blood vessels to increase the volume of blood sent to the penis by nearly eight times. As the penis begins to swell with blood, the swelling causes valves in the veins leaving the penis to shut and thus prevent the blood from exiting. At first the penis becomes enlarged (*tumescent*). As the pressure builds, the penis becomes rigid (*engorged*).

The man generally needs to be in good health in order to have the vigor and desire for sexual activity. However, no matter what his desire, several "mechanical" processes must work before this sequence of events can take place:

The *nerves* must be intact to send the signals from the brain to the blood vessels;

the *large blood vessels* (arteries) must be capable of handling the blood flow into and through the penis;

the *small blood vessels* within the penis must be able to accommodate the additional blood flow; and

the *valves in the veins* leaving the penis must be able to close to trap the blood in the penis.

We are not certain of the exact role the male hormone, testosterone, plays in the erection process, as some men who have been castrated surgically or by an injury can have erections (testosterone can be supplied from other parts of the body). We do know, however, that certain hormonal imbalances, when corrected, can restore potency. But more about that later.

Because the three main "players" are the brain, the nerves to the penis, and the penile blood supply, many of the diagnostic tests focus on the ability of these systems to function.

THE BASIC DIAGNOSTIC WORKUP

Our physician advisors tell us that most men should expect to receive a diagnosis within three visits. On an average, visits are a week apart, allowing, for example, for the return of test results. And on your third visit, your urologist should be able to offer you a choice of several treatment options.

The First Visit

During the first visit your urologist should do the following:

Take your medical history;
take your urological history;
take your sexual history;
perform an examination to assess your general health;
perform a urological physical examination; and
order blood-chemistry tests to check your general health, liver function, kidney function, hormonal balance, blood sugar, and so forth.
Optional: Order a psychological evaluation from a mental-health professional.

When you give your urologist your medical history, he or she will be looking for clues that indicate if you have vascular (blood flow) or neurological (nerve) problems. For example, if you report having shortness of breath upon exertion or if you have had bypass surgery, these may be clues that the arteries to your penis may also have blockage, thus preventing penile engorgement. If you report that you have consumed significant amounts of alcohol over a period of time, this may give your doctor concern about liver function and nerve damage. In addition, your doctor will want to know the names of all prescriptions, over-the-counter, and street drugs you are taking. Sometimes impotence can be corrected by changing to a different medication or by eliminating substances like the nicotine ingested from smoking cigarettes.

Your urological history may reveal that you had prostate, bladder, or pelvic surgery, which may have damaged the nerves or blood vessels supplying the penis. If you have a problem with incontinence, your doctor will want to check out these problems too.

Your sexual history may give your doctor a number

of clues about your condition. For example, if the onset of your impotence problem was *sudden,* and not associated with an injury or surgery, then the problem may be psychogenic. The doctor may ask you if you can gain and keep an erection when you masturbate. For if you can, you probably do not have a physical impotence problem. The physician may then question you about the circumstances immediately preceding the onset, perhaps revealing an unpleasant sexual experience. Further tests will be needed, however, to confirm a psychogenic origin.

If the onset of your impotence was *gradual,* the physician will be more likely to suspect a degenerating physical process. If you report that your penis becomes enlarged but does not become stiff or if your erection lasts only a short time, then the physician may suspect that the valves are leaking blood through the veins. If you report a loss of body hair and sexual libido, the doctor may suspect low testosterone levels.

After taking your history, the urologist specialist will check you over from head to toe, ordering X rays, cardiograms, blood tests, and other standard tests to assess your general health. In addition, the physician will recommend one of several sleep studies (see below).

Some physicians will also refer you to a mental-health professional for a psychological evaluation. We suggest that you do this as we find that virtually every man experiencing impotence—no matter what the origin—has some emotional problems. One of our I.A. chapter urologist medical advisors told us, "I've learned through experience to be concerned about men who are trying to hide things, who seem overly preoccupied with minutiae, who are concerned about how big their penis will be after an implant, or who wonder if an implant will make them a better lover than they were before." He went on to say, "It's not up to me to make a judgment or moral decision about who should or shouldn't receive my services. However, I want the patient to have as positive an experience as possible. Sometimes counseling early on will avoid problems down the road."

Home sleep tests. Every boy and man has periodic, naturally occurring erections during the night. These erections occur during REM (rapid eye movement) sleep, which has been associated with the stage of sleep during which dreams occur. These erections occur in response to biological rhythms regulated by the brain and cannot normally be suppressed. You may have awakened with an erection in the past.

During waking hours, higher-level brain functions (logic, anxiety, fear, and so forth) may suppress these erections. During sleep, however, the higher brain functions are off duty, so to speak, allowing the natural cycles to operate unhampered. The *Snap Gauge* is a simple home test you can use to see if you are responding to these natural body rhythms. The Snap Gauge is equipped with three colored bands that break at three different pressure levels. At bedtime the man slips the Snap Gauge comfortably around his penis. If he has an erection during his sleep, his enlarged penis will break one or more of the colored rings indicating minimal, moderate, or maximum pressure (rigidity).

The Snap Gauge, however, tells the doctor only that you had one erection of unknown duration. It does not say if you had multiple erections or how long your erection lasted. Several nights with no results, however, probably indicate that you have an organic problem that is preventing your penis from responding to your hormonal rhythms; or that your hormonal system is not working properly. This result will require further investigation to pinpoint the cause of the problem.

The nocturnal penile tumescence (NPT) study is a very simple test, and in most situations it can be done in the privacy of your home. Rubber-band-like strain gauges are placed around the penis at the base and just below the head *(glans).* The gauges are connected to a monitor (similar to an electrocardiogram monitor). The test is usually done over a two- or three-night period. The physician can then look at the recordings produced by these studies and usually differentiate between physical and psychological causes of impotence.

NPT studies are a more sophisticated method of monitoring the occurrence of sleep erections. Studies can be undertaken at home or in sleep labs and tell considerably more than the Snap Gauge: number of erections, duration/intensity of tumescence, and frequency intervals are measured using a mercury string gauge with loops at the base and below the head of the penis. A study with normal findings is highly suggestive of psychological impotence. A study showing a decrease in any of the variables most likely reflects a physical cause.

Recently an NPT machine known as the Rigiscan has not only helped physicians determine tumescence but has also revealed that 15 percent of men who have normal tumescence will not achieve full rigidity. Sometimes the partner can report this fact as well. The woman will report that the penis, though enlarged, is not sufficiently stiff to achieve penetration. This is sometimes referred to as a *buckling* phenomenon.

Second Visit and Formal Sleep Studies

At your second visit, your urologist should tell you the results of the tests conducted during your physical examination. If the physical examination and diagnostic tests revealed a health problem, such as diabetes or heart or liver disease, for example, your doctor may refer you to a specialist for further studies and treatment.

For example, Gene, a policeman we spoke with at an

I.A. meeting, said his urologist found a large amount of sugar in his urine. So he referred him to an endocrinologist who could treat the diabetes. Gene said that within a month of getting his diabetes under control, his potency returned. This man was lucky because his early action apparently prevented any permanent damage to nerves or blood vessels.

At the second visit, you should also report the results of your home Snap Gauge tests. Depending on the results, your doctor may recommend a sleep study performed over two to three nights at your home or at a special laboratory. The measurements taken during these tests will further refine the data you gathered during the Snap Gauge tests. Some physicians are bypassing the Snap Gauge test and perform the NPT or Rigiscan tests directly.

Though these tests can be rather expensive, they will provide definitive proof about your physical ability to have good-quality, "natural" erections.

We remember Dean, a man who called us and said, "I paid $75 for a basic visit and he scheduled me for surgery." If your doctor recommends surgery at the second visit, you should be concerned about the thoroughness of the diagnostic procedures. While a doctor may suspect that surgery will be the answer, more testing should be done before that recommendation is made or acted on.

Third Visit: Diagnosis and Recommendations

By your third visit your physician should be able to tell you if your impotence is physically or psychologically based. If you have psychogenic impotence, you should be referred for counseling. The pharmacological erection program (PEP) may also be suggested as a treatment. (See Chapters 8 and 9, which discuss the diagnosis and treatment of psychogenic impotence.)

If you have an organic problem, your physician may recommend treatment options or recommend further tests to pinpoint the specific cause.

BEYOND THE BASICS: PINPOINTING THE PHYSICAL PROBLEM

Even though you may learn that you have a physical problem, the exact reason for your impotence may not be apparent. Until that mystery is revealed, your urologist probably won't recommend treatment. A number of other tests are available to confirm the exact diagnosis. These additional tests should require no more than two to three more visits to complete, thus extending the total time for your diagnosis to probably no more than six weeks.

The following tests will help your physician recommend the best treatment for your particular situation. Usually a blood test is followed by a sleep test (when used) and a Doppler test. Other tests are used as required.

Penile temperature. A thermometer placed in the *urethra* (opening in the penis for urination) will measure the temperature inside the penis. This will help tell the doctor if you have normal penile blood flow. A lower-than-normal reading may indicate arterial blockage. A penile temperature of 1.6 degrees Fahrenheit or more below your body temperature may indicate poor blood flow to the penis.

Cystometrogram. This test detects if the penis is receiving "messages" through the nerves from the brain by measuring the function of the urinary bladder. If the nerves to the bladder are working correctly and the cystometrogram is normal, the nerves to the penis are most likely to be normal. This test is not used much anymore as there are more sophisticated tests available.

Pudendal nerve conduction time. The pudendal nerve is a main nerve to the penis, which has a sensory and motion function. During this test, the penis is stimulated by a mild electrical current for a long enough period to cause contraction of the anal muscles. The test measures the length of time required to stimulate this contraction. This determines whether or not the pudendal nerve serving the penis is intact.

Papaverine/Regitine injection. A papaverine/Regitine (phentolamine mesylate) injection will demonstrate beyond a doubt if your penile vascular system is functioning properly. This test is relatively simple to perform, causes minimal discomfort, and can be performed in the doctor's office. When injected at the base of the penis, the medication will cause an erection within fifteen to twenty minutes. If your vascular system is working, the erection will last from one to four hours.

If there is no rigidity or if your erection lasts for fewer than thirty minutes, the results are suggestive of a venous valve problem. This can be confirmed by injecting a dye into the penis and watching the course of the dye as it leaves the penis *(cavernosagram).* X rays are taken to track the rate of flow.

If the erection is partial or weak, the results may indicate that clogged blood vessels leading to or within the penis are restricting the blood flow to the penis.

Duplex ultrasound scanning machine. This test measures exact blood vessel size and blood flow through the very small penile arteries. A very sensitive noninvasive diagnostic test that is used when an erection is poor or short-lived, perhaps indicating blood "leakage."

Some physicians are using the papaverine/Regitine injection as an early diagnostic tool because if you fail to get an erection, you probably have a vascular problem. Finding the appropriate dosage level, however, may require a couple of tries before the injection works.

Doppler blood-flow studies. A Doppler stethoscope uses ultrasound to detect blood flow in the penis. If this test indicates that blockage exists in the large or medium-size vessels, the doctor may order an angiogram or radionucleotide study to confirm the exact location and nature of the blockage. The ratio of penile blood pressure to arm blood pressure should be larger than 70 percent (0.7).

Radio immunoassay (RIA). This blood test measures testosterone levels most accurately. Time of day the test is taken can greatly affect results as levels are twice as high in early morning as in late afternoon.

Angiogram/angiography. This test should be performed only after the Doppler stethoscope indicates a blood-flow problem in large or medium-size vessels. The angiogram will locate specific blood-vessel blockage and thus indicate if the problem can be corrected surgically.

The doctor inserts a small plastic tube *(catheter)* into a large blood vessel in the leg. Under X-ray control, the doctor threads the tube through the artery and into the large vessel entering the penis. A dye is injected, and X rays are taken to visualize the large and small vessels in the penis. This hospital procedure performed under local anesthetic will help the doctor decide if surgery will be effective in removing the blockage.

Radionucleotide penogram. This relatively new blood-flow test is less invasive than the angiogram. The doctor injects a tiny amount of radioactive "dye" into any vein in the body. Then after a short time the doctor uses a Geiger counter to take a "picture" of the blood flowing through the vessels in the penis. Areas with poor blood flow will contain less "dye" than areas with better flow.

Minnesota Multiphase Personality Inventory (MMPI). This is a psychological evaluation test.

LEARNING THE ANSWERS

"When Bruce went through his diagnostic testing, we knew very little about what to expect," Eileen told the I.A. group. "We didn't even know the right questions to ask. When the doctor discovered irreversible nerve and blood-vessel damage caused by Bruce's diabetes, he offered one solution—a penile implant.

"Bruce had to tell *me* about it. I was furious at being left out. I wanted to know more about this strange thing inside him that was going to be used on *me.* I had the right to know more about it *from the physician.* Now I know that I should have stood up for my rights. After all, we were paying the bill.

"Since then, I've learned that the doctor's word isn't law," she added. "Your urologist should explain the results of your tests, and explain why he or she recommends you take certain actions. You have a right to know."

Our medical advisors tell us that they want to see the partner at least once; and if that's not possible, to talk with her on the telephone. In fact, urologist Dr. Myron Murdock said, "If the man does not want to bring his partner in, I become concerned about what else might be going on."

One of our I.A. chapter Urologist Medical Advisors said that one woman he spoke with objected to the blood-vessel surgery because she was concerned about her husband's health. Pam didn't want him to go through the pain of surgery. Once the doctor assured her that the surgery would not cause a lot of pain and that her husband would receive pain medication, Pam was relieved. The I-Anon chapter members whose husbands had had the surgery also helped allay her fears.

We believe that a man should decide whether or not he wants treatment for his impotence. He has the right to remain chronically impotent if he chooses. In addition, he has the right to choose the recommended medical treatment best suited for him.

Some men choose one form of treatment for a while and then switch to another. For example, Ed, a recently widowed man we talked with at an I.A. meeting, decided to try injection therapy because he wasn't sure he wanted to rejoin the sex scene. Later we learned that Ed met a very nice woman whom he wished to marry. At that time Ed went ahead with implant surgery.

We're getting ahead of our story though. First let's look at the many different medical conditions that can cause chronic impotence, and how each of these conditions can be treated.

5

MEDICAL PROBLEMS: THE VASCULAR SYSTEM

Impotence is usually *not* a primary ailment. It is a symptom of something else. That "something else" may be a serious medical problem—even a life-threatening one. Therefore, you should not delay consulting with a urologist specialist to determine the cause of your impotence. And, with today's options, there's almost no reason why you should not be able to overcome the effects of your impotence, if you so choose.

In this chapter and the next, we shall explain how toxic substances, medications, hormonal imbalances, injuries, surgeries, and chronic illnesses such as diabetes, arteriosclerosis, and heart and liver disease can "show up" as impotence. In addition, we will tell you the recommended treatment for each disorder.

Chapter 7, "Overcoming the Effects of Impotence," describes in more detail the treatments available for men when Mother Nature can no longer do it alone.

A SHORT LESSON IN ANATOMY

When a man becomes sexually aroused by his senses—sight, taste, touch—or thoughts, signals travel from his brain down his spinal cord to nerves in the pelvis. The signals continue their journey through the pelvic nerves that travel parallel to the arteries supplying the penis. This nervous activity causes these arteries to dilate, sending a surge of blood into the penis. Simultaneously valves (*polsters*) on the return (venous) side (located in tissue next to arteries) close so blood cannot leave the penis. The spongy tissue inside the penis engorges with blood, causing the penis to get bigger and harder. The man has an erection.

The penis contains three rodlike structures. The two spongy structures on the top of the penis (*corpora cavernosa*) trap the blood for the erection. The third rod (*corpus spongiosum*) located in the middle and beneath the urethra also becomes erect; however, it is primarily filled by the urethra. The tip or head of the penis (*glans penis*) is part of the corpus spongiosum.

The blood supplies for the three rodlike bodies are separate: right and left corpora cavernosa and corpus spongiosum. In addition, the right and left corpora cavernosa share a common connecting channel through which blood can flow. The interruption of this blood supply may account for 60 to 70 percent of all impotence.

MEDICAL PROBLEMS CAUSING VASCULAR DISEASE

Diabetes

Diabetes is the number-one cause of chronic impotence. There are an estimated 13 million diabetic men in the

United States. And at least 50 percent of all diabetic men will develop impotence in their lifetime. One-third of thirty-year-old diabetic men are impotent.

You should not simply assume, however, that because you are diabetic, your impotence is due to a physical problem. For example, Jeff had suffered a stroke, he took high blood pressure medication, and he had a family history of diabetes and coronary artery disease. But a sleep test showed that Jeff was psychogenically impotent. In contrast, Eric, a young diabetic who experienced abrupt onset of organic impotence, had difficulty getting proper medical attention because his doctors thought it was "all in his head."

Eighty percent of diabetic men suffer from premature hardening of the arteries, especially of the small vessels in the penis. The restricted penile blood supply not only hampers the engorgement process, it also damages the nerves leading to the penis. The severity of the diabetes does not seem to have a relationship to the effects on impotence: for example, Frankie, a mild diabetic, suffered total impotence; whereas Alec, a severe diabetic, had no problem at all.

The diagnosis of diabetes can be made by urinalysis and blood tests. In some cases, bringing previously uncontrolled diabetes under control through diet or insulin therapy will restore potency.

Dale, a mildly diabetic policeman who came to one of our I.A. chapter meetings, brought his impotence under control by changing his diet. (He cut out all sugar other than natural sugars, increased his fiber intake, and reduced his fat and cholesterol consumption.) In cases where irreversible blood-vessel and nerve damage has occurred—as with Jim—a man should consider trying an external management device that can increase the blood in the penis. Or he should get an inflatable penile implant, as did Fred, a diabetic who was also an alcoholic. Chapter

7 contains more about the treatment for overcoming the effects of chronic impotence.

Hardening of the Arteries

Hardening of the arteries, the leading physical deterioration resulting in impotence, is more common in people who are obese, diabetic, hypertensive, or who smoke. Hardening of the arteries can be diagnosed a number of ways.

When taking the history, the doctor looks for a number of key points: a history of high blood pressure, hypertension, and heart disease, for example. The doctor may suspect this condition if, as Mel did, you report that you get pains in your legs, thighs, and buttocks during physical activity.

On examination, the doctor may find decreased or unequal pulses in the lower extremities, an enlarged *aorta* (main artery leading from the heart to the lower extremities), or irregular noises created by blood flowing through rough blood vessels coated with an obstructive fatty material (*plaque*).

The man may complain that he has poor erections: They are infrequent or not stiff enough. Or he may complain that he "loses it" in the middle of lovemaking. Richard reported to his urologist that he had trouble maintaining his erection when using particular coital positions, especially when he was on top (the missionary position). His difficulty probably had more to do with the strenuousness of his effort in this position. What Richard described is what is commonly called the *steal syndrome* because his restricted blood supply—further limited by strenuous physical activity—was "stealing" blood away from his penis. When his doctor told him to change from the missionary position to lying on his back or side, to avoid the large muscle activity at his hips, Richard did much better.

The doctor can confirm arteriosclerosis with a Doppler stethoscope and urethral temperature study. A lower-than-normal urethral temperature indicates impaired blood flow in the penis. A Doppler study will reveal if there is blockage in the large to medium-size blood vessels in the penis. If the Doppler study is normal but there is a lowered penile temperature, then the disease probably involves the small vessels (under 4 to 5 millimeters in diameter—a fraction of an inch) in the penis.

From the beginning of Howard's second marriage, he had a problem with impotence. He'd had coronary bypass surgery several years before and he had a family history of hypertension and heart disease. A medical workup revealed that he had mild Peyronie's disease (see below), and in his sleep test he had no good-quality, sustained nocturnal erections. Further diagnostic tests revealed chronic *vasculogenic* (inhibited blood flow) impotence. After attending a few I.A. meetings and talking about his problem with others experiencing similar difficulties, Howard decided to get a penile implant.

Vascular surgery and *vasodilators* (medications that help blood vessels to expand) are used to improve penile blood flow. We shall discuss the pros and cons of each later in this chapter.

Heart Disease

Heart disease is usually associated with vascular disease: hardening of the arteries. Severe heart disease, however, may lower heart output so much that even a "healthy" penis cannot get enough blood to engorge. In such cases, the urologist should work closely with the cardiologist to control the heart disease. Should circulation remain poor, however, the impotence may have to be resolved using an implant or external management device.

Peyronie's Disease

Peyronie's disease is very common among men from forty to sixty years old, and especially among men who are heavy drinkers. Our Urologist Medical Advisors tell us that they see several cases each month. Peyronie's disease is the deposition of scar tissue in the shaft of the penis, probably due to the inflammation of blood vessels in the penis. Diabetics and people with rheumatoid arthritis or fibrosing diseases involving other organs tend to have a higher incidence of this condition. Many men affected by Peyronie's disease become extremely anxious, fearing that they have cancer, which usually is not the case.

Often the inflammation follows some traumatic incident with the penis—sex itself, for example, which incites inflammation of the arteries and veins in the penis. And when the inflammation subsides, scar tissue is left in the vessels. Initially the man complains of pain. But then the pain goes away and he is left with a thickening in the shaft of the penis, usually at the top and toward the base. When he has an erection, the penis curves toward this thickened tissue. The curvature occurs because the scar tissue will not stretch and allow the penis to expand fully, the fibrous plaque (usually nonmalignant growths; a form of scar tissue) tethers the penis.

Aaron reported that he would get an excellent erection up to the plaque, but beyond that point his penis was soft, making vaginal entry difficult. This is a common complaint.

Within a year, 90 percent of men with Peyronie's disease will improve spontaneously. Often the physician will recommend waiting at least one year before treating the disorder. Although the thickness never really goes away, the curvature may improve. Various treatments including ultrasound, steroid injections, vitamin E, and a medication called Potaba have been used with poor results. Some physicians inject enzymes that will "digest" or dissolve the scar tissue; however, this is still an experimental procedure.

If the curvature is severe—a condition affecting 30 percent of those with Peyronie's disease—and the man is still potent, surgery may be considered. Surgical removal of the plaque runs a high risk of damaging the nerves in the penis—thus causing it to go permanently numb. When this happens, it is very difficult to have sex.

Ten percent of men with Peyronie's disease will develop severe symptoms, including blood-vessel obstruction in the walls of the corpora midway along the shaft of the penis. This severe and painful curvature usually prevents sexual activity and often causes impotence. This condition may be corrected by either removing (excising) or cutting slits into (incising) the plaque (so it will lie flat) and inserting an implant on top of it into the penis.

Priapism

Sometimes damage to the valves (polsters) in the veins leaving the penis can cause an unwanted, sustained, and painful erection, known as priapism. The erection may last for many hours or even days. A sustained erection can cause *fibrosis* (scar tissue) and damage to the fine structures of the spongy corpora of the penis and cause further damage to the valves. With repeated episodes, the valves may become incapable of trapping the blood in the penis and the man may become impotent.

Priapism is associated with certain blood disorders such as sickle-cell anemia, leukemia, and other blood cancers. In addition, chemotherapy can cause a sludging effect in the blood, increasing its blood thickness (*viscosity*). When this happens, the blood clots and becomes trapped in the erectile chambers.

Priapism can and should be treated promptly by a

physician, who will drain the blood from the penis and reduce the pressure on the structures. If this is not done, the lack of blood flow and oxygen to the penis will cause extensive scarring and may destroy the erectile chambers so they can no longer respond as they should. Continued problems with this disorder almost always require using a penile implant.

Aneurysm of the Penis

An *aneurysm,* or bulging of a blood vessel, of the penis does not cause impotence but may be a signal that conditions favoring impotence are developing. An aneurysm is usually caused by hardening of the arteries or by trauma to the penis itself. If left untreated, the weak spot may rupture.

Venogenic Impotence

Venogenic impotence accounts for many cases of "unexplained" impotence, which up until now were mistakenly attributed to psychological causes. Venogenic impotence occurs most frequently in young or middle-age men who have no recognized risk factors such as diabetes or hypertension.

In the normal erection, blood flows into the penis and is trapped in the corpora cavernosa. The polsters in the veins leaving the penis shut tight to provide a seal. In venogenic impotence, these valves leak, allowing the blood to escape before intercourse is complete. You might think of this as trying to blow up a balloon that has a hole in it. Some men, such as Clifford, reported that their penis never achieved full rigidity so they could gain penetration. Others, such as Martin, said that they got a good erection, but lost it in a few minutes.

Several tests are used to diagnose this problem. First the urologist will confirm that blood flow to the penis is normal with Doppler ultrasound. Then the physician will administer an injection of papaverine and/or papaverine and Regitine to stimulate blood flow to the penis. With damaged valves, the man will obtain a poor erection, implying that the blood is rapidly "leaking" out.

If this occurs, the urologist then will use the duplex ultrasound scanning machine to measure exact blood-vessel size and blood flow. To confirm the exact location of the leakage, the doctor will then order the penile cavernosogram. This is an outpatient test and causes minimal discomfort.

Surgery to restrict venous flow from the penis is quite often successful unlike arterial surgery, which tends to have a poor outcome. (See Surgical Repair for Polsters, p. 62.)

TREATMENT FOR VASCULAR PROBLEMS

Blood Vessel (Arterial) Surgery

The surgeon has several options for opening or clearing out clogged large to medium-size arteries.

With the *endarterectomy,* the surgeon opens an artery, removes the plaque and damaged portion of the vessel, and reconnects the artery. With impotence, usually both sides of the penis will be involved. However, repairing one side will frequently produce sufficient blood to restore potency. Only on rare occasions must both sides of the penis be operated on.

The surgeon may decide to use another vein or artery to *bypass* the area of obstruction.

In addition, the surgeon can *revascularize* the area by bringing an artery from another area to the penis and connecting the good artery directly into the spongy tissue of the penis. The transplanted artery will even produce small sprouts into the penis and thus significantly improve the blood supply. Surgeons report that they get excellent long-term results with this procedure, especially with men who have suffered from a traumatic pelvic injury that damaged the pudendal artery in the pelvis.

The surgeon can also use *balloon angioplasty* to displace the obstruction. The surgeon inserts a deflated balloon through the arteries to the point of blockage. The balloon is then inflated to compress the plaque against the arterial wall and open the passage.

Blood-vessel surgery to remove plaque can produce spectacular results in the short run. However, usually within six months to a year, the vessel again will become clogged and the man will become impotent once more. Initially, 50 to 60 percent of men will respond favorably to this procedure. After one year, however, only 10 percent are still potent. This is because their vascular disease is becoming progressively worse, or because the narrowed vascular branches are creating too much resistance, causing clotting and blocking in the pathways further on. Because of this, less and less reconstructive vascular surgery is being done.

The best candidates for vascular surgery are young patients who do not have diabetes or blood-vessel disease. Patients must realize that they have a poor chance of good long-term erectile function, and they should be prepared to undergo a second surgical procedure to insert an implant should the vascular surgery fail.

Surgical Repair for Polsters (Valves)

The surgeon can tie off the veins containing leaking valves to obstruct or increase the resistance to the venous outflow. There are no good statistics on the success rates for this procedure. However, because this is a fairly easy operation, and because there is some chance it will improve potency, the operation may be worthwhile. (See Venogenic Impotence, p. 60.)

Vasodilators

If the small vessels are involved, they may be dilated with oral medication or with penile (papaverine/Regitine) injections. Vasodilators work well with partially impotent men and with cigarette smokers. Dan reported remarkable improvement with this medication. Over 50 percent report satisfactory improvement. The physician may also recommend blood thinners, including a daily low-dose aspirin regimen, to improve blood flow. If the man does not respond to vasodilators, the physician may recommend an aphrodisiac (see Chapter 7, Aphrodisiacs, p. 81).

Vasoactive Intestinal Peptide (VIP)

Vasoactive intestinal peptide, or VIP, consists of a group of amino acids that triggers nerve transmitters at nerve endings, thereby increasing blood flow. It is now believed that results of this stimulation are the ultimate transmitter of blood to the penis. It is expected that medication to be taken by injection or orally to stimulate blood flow to the penis will be developed soon.

As you know, impotence may be the side effect of a serious underlying medical problem. The symptoms should not be ignored. If your impotence cannot be corrected with vascular surgery or by vasodilators, however, there is no reason for despair. A number of other options are available to you. You *can* have a satisfying sex life. Chapters 6 and 7 will help you understand more about impotence and about overcoming the effects of impotence.

6

MEDICAL PROBLEMS: THE NERVOUS SYSTEM

The nerves supplying the blood vessels leading to the penis and the nerves supplying the penis itself are vital to potency. Nerves can be impaired or damaged from disease, injury, surgery, radiation exposure, and by toxic substances. In this chapter we shall familiarize you with these conditions and with the treatment available for them.

NERVE DAMAGE

Spinal Cord Injury

Spinal cord injury does not always cause impotence. The nerve centers for erection are located in the *sacral* (lower) section of the spinal cord. If the cord is severed above this nerve center, emotionally stimulated erections cannot occur.

A paraplegic or quadriplegic whose spine is completely severed may still have good reflex action in response to direct stroking of the penis. This erection will continue as long as the penis is physically stimulated.

Impotence problems often occur with individuals who have suffered partial injuries to the spinal cord. It seems that when the nerves can transmit messages from the brain to the penis, these impulses may actually interfere with the natural reflex phenomenon. Men who suffer damage to the erectile nerve center located in the sacral section of the cord usually lose the natural reflex action.

Bobby, a very nice young man who'd been injured on the job, asked us for assistance. His injury had left him a quadriplegic who was able to manipulate his shoulders somewhat. He had a very understanding partner who was willing to help him. Because his hand movement was impaired, the couple wanted to get an inflatable implant that she could operate. After his surgery, they wrote us and said they were both very happy with the results.

Many spinal cord injury victims choose to get a penile implant because they are easy to use, even by the partner.

Other Diseases Affecting the Nerves

Multiple sclerosis (MS) is a degenerative disease that destroys the insulating sheath around the nerves. Men with this disease complain of weakness in their extremities as well as difficulties with their bowel, urinary, and erectile functions. When the nerves supplying the penis or blood vessels to the penis become involved, MS may cause impotence. (Note: Muscular dystrophy, a degenerative muscle disease, does *not* cause impotence.)

Amyotrophic lateral sclerosis, tumors of the spinal

cord and brain, and strokes all have the potential for causing impotence. Diabetes often causes nerve damage (*neuropathy*) by restricting the blood supply to the nerves.

Poisoning from heavy metals such as lead may also cause nerve damage resulting in impotence.

Pelvic Trauma

Approximately one-third of severe pelvic fractures interrupt the blood supply to the penis or to the nerves supplying the penis.

Pelvic nerves can be injured in a number of ways: pelvic fracture from an accident, bleeding into the pelvis, war injuries, gun accidents, and so forth. If the blood supply to the testicles (*testes*), which produce the male hormone, is disrupted, the affected testicle(s) may be destroyed and require surgical removal.

With modern microsurgical techniques, sometimes surgeons can reconnect severed nerves. In time, the nerves will reestablish the path from the brain to penis and potency will be restored. If the damage is too extensive, however, surgeons may not be able to restore the nerve pathways.

Dennis was injured in a hunting accident. He was fortunate enough to be treated at a hospital with a very fine neurological surgical team who restored the nerve connection to his penis. After several months he began to get some feeling again. Eventually the nerves grew back and his potency returned.

Should the testicles be damaged, testosterone replacement therapy will help restore libido and maintain sexual performance.

If the impotence persists, the man may consider the use of injections, external management devices, or an implant.

Radical Cancer Surgery/ Radiation Therapy

Radical surgery to remove cancers of the bladder, prostate, colon, rectum, or anus may destroy nerves and blood vessels supplying the penis. In addition, radiation therapy for treating cancers of the pelvic area, bladder, and prostate, and for treating Hodgkin's disease and lymphoma may injure pelvic nerves and penile blood supply. Forty percent of men receiving radiation treatment for prostate cancer will experience decreased erectile function.

Sidney was told by his surgeon that his radical cancer surgery would make him impotent. At the time, though, his primary concern was saving his life from the deadly disease. When he was recovering, his impotence didn't bother him. However, when he felt like having relations with his wife again, Sidney was devastated. He told us that if he'd had a gun in the house he would have shot himself. Fortunately the couple sought help, and now that Sidney has his implant they are both very happy.

Dr. Patrick Walsh at the Department of Neurology of Johns Hopkins University Hospital has developed a procedure for removing a cancerous prostate without causing impotence for 60 to 70 percent of patients. There is some concern that this procedure may not be removing enough tissue to prevent the cancer from recurring. It will take ten to fifteen years to demonstrate if it is a viable cancer operation.

These radical cancer surgeries should be distinguished from partial or complete surgery for benign (noncancerous) prostate disease. The TUR (transurethral resection of the prostate) procedure performed to improve urination *should not cause impotence.* (Note: TUR may cause retrograde ejaculation, where the semen squirts into the bladder instead of out the penis and is voided during the next urination without any ill effects.)

These days not nearly so many people are becoming impotent from radical colon surgery because of newer surgical techniques that require the removal of less tissue. This is in contrast to colostomy patients of many years ago who almost always were impotent following surgery. Many colostomy patients do, however, experience a great deal of emotional stress from the change that occurs in their body image. Even the mechanics of the appliances used to collect normal body fluids produces emotional strain. Many have found the support from the Ostomy Association very helpful. For those who become impotent, external management devices or penile implants can restore satisfactory sexual performance. More about this in Chapter 7.

Kidney Disease

Renal failure has no direct effect on impotence. However, 50 percent of men with kidney failure experience impotence. Hemodialysis, a procedure used to remove toxic wastes from the blood, apparently leaves some toxic materials in the blood that affect the nerves supplying the penis. In addition, antihypertensive medications taken to improve renal function may cause impotence. Papaverine/Regitine injection therapy may not be recommended for these patients because these drugs may adversely affect the kidney.

For no apparent reason, Gil's kidneys began to fail when he was only fifty years old. At first he received antihypertensive medication to improve his kidney function. Soon after beginning the drug, he began experiencing erectile problems. His doctor altered his medication; this helped for a while, but with further deterioration in his kidney function, Gil had to go on dialysis, which made him totally impotent. Fortunately, Gil received a kidney transplant. When his normal renal function resumed, so did his potency.

TOXIC SUBSTANCES—MEDICATIONS, NICOTINE, AND ALCOHOL

When ingested into the body, a number of substances can impair the blood supply to the penis and/or cause nerve damage.

- Medications, especially those for hypertension
  - Tranquilizers
  - Muscle relaxants
- Over-the-counter medications
  - Decongestants
  - Nasal sprays
  - Antihistamines
- Nicotine from cigarette smoking
- Alcohol
- Drug abuse

Medications

A number of medications—prescription and over-the-counter drugs—can cause penile blood-flow problems, affect blood pressure, and alter the body's neurologic status. The chief offenders are tranquilizers, muscle relaxants, antihistamines, and medications that control blood pressure. Over-the-counter drugs such as nasal decongestants, nasal sprays, sinus medication, antihistamines, and low back strain medications can also contribute to impotence.

One of the most popular drugs prescribed today is Tagamet (cimetidine), for the treatment of ulcers. However, Tagamet can lower sexual desire and cause impotence.

One urologist told us a particularly interesting story about a man whom he had referred to an ear, nose, and throat specialist to cure his impotence. The man had been using an antihistamine nose spray for years. Once the specialist got him off the spray, his impotence disappeared.

Often the medication can be changed or the dosage adjusted to relieve the impotence problem.

SOME MEDICATIONS THAT CAN CAUSE IMPOTENCE
(lists are ever-changing; here are just a few)

BRAND NAME	GENERIC NAME
Aldactone, Aldactazide	spironolactone
Aldoril, Aldomet, Aldoclor	methyldopa
Combipres, Catapres	clonidine hydrochloride
Diupres, Regroton, Demi-Regroton	reserpine
Eutonyl	pargyline hydrochloride
Hygroton, Regroton, Combipres	chlorthalidone
Ismelin	guanethidine sulfate
Premarin	estrogen
Serpasil, Hydropres	reserpine
Serpentina, Raudixin, Harmonyl	rauwolfia
Tagamet	cimetidine

Nicotine

The nicotine ingested from cigarette smoking is a poison, a potent *vasoconstrictor* that decreases the size of blood vessels. Although nicotine is not likely to create an impotence problem, it certainly can add to another underlying cause and make the impotence worse. Discontinuing the smoking and using vasodilators often can significantly improve the situation.

Neil, a heavy smoker, called us one day terrified because his urologist had recommended that he get an implant. After discussing his problems with us, Neil decided to get a second opinion. The urologist specialist we referred him to could find no severe medical problems other than a vascular restriction. So he recommended that Neil stop smoking and take a vasodilator to dilate the blood vessels serving his penis. Neil followed the urologist's advice and he and his wife soon resumed a normal sex life. Although the results Neil obtained were rare, it's often worth a try.

Alcohol

Ingesting alcohol over a prolonged period of time may cause nerve damage, premature hardening of the arteries, and liver disease, each of which may cause impotence. In addition, alcohol may create emotional tension and difficulties between the partners and in this way indirectly affect potency. (See also Chapter 5, section on Hardening of the Arteries, pp. 56–57.)

In alcoholics with liver disease a protein that binds with testosterone is produced, so it does not perform its usual function. Some physicians will try testosterone supplements with these men to see if it will help. If there is no improvement within three to six weeks, there probably won't be.

After consulting a urologist specialist, Perry decided to get an implant. He failed, however, to tell his doctor that he was an alcoholic. When Perry's son, a medical technician who worked in the hospital where the urologist practiced, learned of his father's omissions, he told the doctor. The doctor canceled Perry's surgery immediately and confronted him with the fact that his drinking could be causing his impotence. Perry decided to give up his drinking, but it was too late: The nerve damage was irreversible. So the doctor rescheduled his implant surgery.

The reason we're sharing this story with you is to emphasize the importance of being completely honest with your doctor. If Perry's potency had returned when he stopped drinking, he could have avoided surgery.

Drug Abuse

All hard drugs—cocaine, heroin, and morphine-based derivatives—can cause impotence. *Marijuana* can contribute to impotence problems in low or moderate dosages, and can cause nerve damage in high dosages or over long-term use.

HORMONAL ABNORMALITIES AND DEFICIENCIES

Normal Body Hormonal Rhythms

Sex-hormone deficiencies account for less than 5 percent of impotence, and low testosterone levels account for 90 percent of these cases. Some background information about how testosterone is produced by the testicles may help you understand what can cause these hormonal problems.

As you may recall, we mentioned earlier that every "normal" man has periodic erections throughout the day and night because of a natural hormonal rhythm controlled by the hypothalamus of the brain. Every ninety minutes or so, the hypothalamus stimulates the pituitary gland located near the base of the brain to produce LH (luteinizing hormone) and FSH (follicle-stimulating hormone). Traveling through the bloodstream to the testes, LH tells these glands to produce testosterone.

Low Testosterone Level

Testosterone regulates your sex drive, maintains your secondary sex characteristics (beard, low voice, pubic hair, and so forth), and—we think—aids with erections. The reason we hedge here is that, as we mentioned earlier, some men who have been castrated—whose testes were removed surgically or by an accident—can continue to have erections *without* taking testosterone supplements.

A testosterone deficiency may occur when any one of the steps in the following cycle breaks down: if the hypothalamus fails to stimulate the pituitary gland; if the pituitary gland fails to produce adequate amounts of LH; or if the testes are unable to respond by producing testosterone.

Howard attended an I.A. meeting and asked if he should be there. He explained that his problem was that he had no desire. The medical advisors—a urologist and psychiatrist team—assured him that he *did* belong. After a medical evaluation, Howard received testosterone therapy from the urologist and counseling from the psychiatrist to help him overcome his low self-esteem. Soon they were able to get Howard back on track to a satisfactory sexual relationship with his wife.

Testosterone replacement therapy is effective for reversing impotence only for men who have significantly low levels of this hormone. Testosterone levels can be measured most accurately with the radio immunoassay (RIA) blood test. Testosterone levels are twice as high at 8:00 A.M., for example, as between 4:00 P.M. and 8:00 P.M. The physician should obtain blood samples both in the morning and in the afternoon. Then readings for both times of day should be compared. If the morning level is the same as the usually lower afternoon level, the deficiency is confirmed.

In addition, the doctor should compare the testosterone reading with the LH and FSH levels. When testosterone is high, LH and FSH should be relatively low. When testosterone is low, LH and FSH should be relatively high, telling the testes to "get with it." If LH and FSH are high and the testes are not responding, the testes may be incapable of making testosterone. Further tests will be needed to confirm the nature of the problem.

Testosterone Replacement Therapy

Testosterone is not an entirely safe drug for men who do not have a documented testosterone deficiency. Men who take it unnecessarily can run a higher risk of getting liver cancer, prostate cancer, chemical hepatitis, severe sodium absorption (water retention), hypertension (high blood pressure), and heart disease. Our medical advisors tell us that testosterone should be given only to patients who have—at the least—a borderline testosterone level.

Oil-based testosterone injections last two to three weeks. One injection isn't enough to prove anything. Only after six weeks of weekly or biweekly injections will you know if the hormone will improve your potency. If the testosterone does work, a maintenance dose taken every four to six weeks should maintain your potency. Oral methyl testosterone is associated with a high incidence of chemical hepatitis and should not be used more than four to six weeks, according to our medical advisors.

Ernest came to an I.A. meeting and told the medical advisor that he'd been taking testosterone for three years with no results. The medical advisor's examination revealed that Ernest had severe vascular problems. No amount of testosterone could have improved Ernest's condition. In fact, Ernest was lucky the testosterone had not caused serious side effects.

Pituitary Tumors

Sometimes a pituitary tumor may interfere with pituitary function. This is usually revealed by a blood test showing that testosterone, LH, and FSH are all low. The testosterone is low because the pituitary is not stimulating the testes to produce testosterone. Often the pituitary tumor causes other abnormalities, such as growth hormone and thyroid hormone deficiencies.

When this problem arises, usually your urologist will refer you to an endocrinologist (hormone specialist) for treatment. Pituitary tumors may be corrected by hormonal therapy consisting of testosterone supplements or sometimes by a combination of testosterone and LH supplements. When testosterone levels are restored to normal, the impotence problem will most probably disappear.

Excess Prolactin

An excess of prolactin may cause impotence in a very small percentage of men. Prolactin is the hormone most commonly associated with nursing (lactating) mothers. Excess prolactin, caused by a pituitary tumor or other abnormalities, causes a decrease in testosterone production. In a very short time, the drug Parlodel (bromocriptine) will shrink the tumor and will reduce prolactin levels. Once testosterone production returns to normal, the impotence problem can be resolved.

Excess Estrogen

Excess estrogen (the female sex hormone) may also suppress testosterone production by suppressing the pituitary gland's LH production. Men with estrogen-producing tumors or men taking estrogen (for prostate cancer, for example) may experience this problem. Also, chronic alcoholics with liver disease cannot metabolize (degrade and change) the normal amounts of estrogen produced by the adrenal glands and testicles. Over time, the estrogens gradually build up and interfere with testosterone production.

There is some evidence that large numbers of fat cells, which occur in extremely obese men, may produce enough estrogen to suppress testosterone production.

OTHER PROBLEMS CAUSING IMPOTENCE

Sickle-cell anemia. Sickle-cell anemia can cause a sludging effect on blood cells. When this happens, blood flow to the penis may become restricted, causing impotence.

Obesity. This is usually not a factor causing physical impotence. Extremely obese people may have self-image problems or may have difficulty participating in coitus because of their size and bulk. (See also Excess Estrogen, p. 75.)

Congenital anomalies (primary impotence). Sometimes the man is born with no spongy (corporal) tissue in the penis. The penis will appear baggy and enlarged. Because he has no erectile tissue, he cannot get an erection. This condition can be treated with an implant. (*Primary impotence* means that from birth the man never functioned sexually. *Secondary impotence* means that the impotence developed sometime after birth.)

Incontinence. Loss of urinary control is not directly related to impotence. However, radical prostate surgery and trauma to the pelvic bone and structures—which lead to urinary incontinence—may also cause impotence. Even if the man is not physically impotent, the embarrassment of incontinence may cause him to avoid lovemaking or to become psychogenically impotent.

Our medical advisors tell us that most physicians will wait three to six months after the initial surgery (radical prostate surgery, for example) to put in an erection device and incontinence device. Some physicians may even wait one year because the incontinence may improve on its own in that time.

Liver disease. See Alcohol, page 71.

Other chronic debilitating disorders. Any chronic debilitating disorder—malignancy, malnutrition, radical chemotherapy, and severe illness—may cause temporary or chronic impotence. If the basic medical disorder can be corrected, the potency may return. If, however, the medical disorder is not reversible, treatment should be considered.

In the next chapter we shall discuss the many options available to men who, because of irreparable nerve or blood-vessel damage, must give Mother Nature an assist. You will discover how nearly every chronically impotent man can overcome the effects of impotence and restore successful lovemaking to his relationship.

7

OVERCOMING THE EFFECTS OF IMPOTENCE

Nearly every man suffering from *irreversible impotence* can enjoy a satisfying sex life if he offers nature a little help through medical treatment, injection therapy, an external management device, or a penile implant. In this chapter we shall discuss the options available to couples who want to overcome the effects of chronic impotence and resume a loving and fulfilling sexual relationship.

MAKING THE "RIGHT" CHOICE

Many couples ask us, "What's the best treatment?" or "Which device works the best?" And quite honestly, we must respond that *the choice of treatment is an issue between the impotent man, his urologist specialist, and his partner.* Our job, and the job of I.A. and I-Anon, is to provide couples with enough information about treatment options that they can ask intelligent questions and make informed decisions about their unique situation. In support of that role, I.A.

and I-Anon provide manufacturer's literature about every medically approved device or treatment to anyone requesting information. All requests are treated with the strictest confidence. (Mail your inquiries to Impotents Anonymous, 119 South Ruth Street, Department Y, Maryville, TN 37801. To find out more about the I.A. and I-Anon organizations, chapters, and services, we recommend you read *Impotents Anonymous* by our National Medical Advisor, Myron I. Murdock, M.D. Copies are available through I.A.)

Choosing the "right" treatment depends on a number of factors:

1. *The diagnosed cause of your chronic impotence*—for example, blood-vessel disease, Peyronie's disease, venous leakage, central nervous system disease, psychogenic problems, and so forth. Injection therapy, for example, would not work well for Perry because his Peyronie's disease caused severe curvature of his penis with resultant pain, and injection therapy would not resolve this difficulty. It was, however, the perfect option for reducing Lee's performance anxiety while he was being counseled for his psychogenic impotence.
2. *The degree to which the impotent man accepts the permanency of his impotence.* If a man believes that with time his potency will return, as Burl did, he will be less likely to consider a permanent treatment such as a penile implant. Burl tried several temporary solutions—injection therapy and using an external management device—as long as he remained in that twilight zone of uncertainty. Once Burl realized that he had a permanent condition, he selected the permanent solution: a penile implant.
3. *Other medical conditions*—for example, liver disease, abnormal heart rhythm (cardiac arrhythmias), high blood pressure, sickle-cell anemia, radiation therapy,

prior surgeries, and so forth. The aphrodisiac yohimbine, for example, was not recommended to Joe, who had a history of high blood pressure, or to Martin, who had cardiac arrhythmia. For these men, an external management device or penile implant was more attractive.

4. *Medications you take*—for example, levodopa (for Parkinson's disease), central nervous system depressants, and morphine-based pain medications. Injection therapy, for example, may interfere with other medications. When this is the case, your physician may recommend an external management device or penile implant.
5. *Cost factors*—including medical, surgical, and hospital expenses as well as insurance coverage. Injection therapy and external management devices may be less expensive options than penile implants. Before making your decision, however, you should consult with your insurance carrier—they are all different. The only way to be sure about what your insurance covers—diagnostic testing, medical treatment, and/or surgery—is to ask before you seek medical treatment.
6. *Personal preferences* of the impotent man *and* of his partner—including feelings about the treatment aesthetics, the amount of time available for surgical recovery, individual tolerance to pain and discomfort, and so forth. We'll address these issues throughout this chapter.

In the discussions of treatment options that follow, you will learn the role each of these factors plays in formulating your doctor's recommendations and in making your personal decision. And you will gain enough understanding about each technique to pursue a personal investigation of your most promising choices.

MEDICAL TREATMENT OPTIONS

Aphrodisiacs (Yohimbine)

How does yohimbine work? American Indians and Africans have known about the effects of yohimbine for centuries. Yohimbine occurs naturally in the bark of evergreen trees. Doctors believe the drug works by improving the performance of the nerves serving the end of the penis. The drug may be effective for men who have failed to respond to vasodilators. Although there have been no large-scale studies to prove the drug's effectiveness, a small percentage of men do report that yohimbine helps.

Who should use yohimbine? Tests suggest that the medication is most effective when the man has mild or moderate impotence, as in Conrad's case. Even though his hormone tests were normal, Conrad complained of low sexual desire and intermittent erection failures. He consulted his urologist after six months. Based on a complete diagnostic workup, the urologist diagnosed a mild bloodflow problem. After three weeks on yohimbine, Conrad's condition improved and no other treatment was required. If the problem has persisted for over five years, studies show that yohimbine will have little or no benefit.

What is the dosage? The usual recommended dose is three tablets daily. However, many patients report improvement with a daily dosage of at least five tablets. Often the effects are cumulative, with satisfactory results obtained after two to three weeks of treatment.

What are the side effects? Potential side effects include excess salivation, increased blood pressure, and increased or abnormal heart rhythm. *Men with heart disease or blood pressure problems should not use yohimbine.* If after six weeks you do not respond to this drug, you should reassess its usefulness with your doctor and consider alternative treatments.

PEP—The Pharmacological Erection Program

Many men who have psychological or organic impotence are looking for a nonsurgical treatment. Various medications, including vasodilating drugs and yohimbine, have been effective for some. The papaverine/Regitine penile injection therapy program (PEP) has produced satisfactory results for a large number of men.

How long has PEP been in use? In Europe, penile injection therapy for the treatment of impotence has been used successfully since the early 1980s. Physicians in the United States, however, have been using this therapy only since the mid-1980s. At the time of this writing, papaverine/Regitine injection therapy has not been approved by the Food and Drug Administration (FDA) for treating impotence, although it is approved for the treatment of hypertension. Doctors, however, can use FDA-approved medications for "unapproved" purposes. Because of this situation, your urologist may request that you sign a consent form before you receive this therapy.

How does PEP work? A simple injection test in the doctor's office will demonstrate whether or not PEP will work for you. The doctor may need to administer test doses to determine your sensitivity to the drug. Then the urologist can mix (titrate) a specially formulated solution that you can self-inject at home.

Within five to fifteen minutes, a single injection directly into the corpus cavernosum at the base of the penis will cause a good erection lasting from one to four hours. The medication is injected with a tuberculin- or insulin-type syringe and needle (26 gauge or smaller). Patients report feeling a small sting.

A number of men, like Dan, think PEP is wonderful. Dan and his partner were thrilled with the quick and consistently good results. Others, like Hank, find the procedure unaesthetic or, after some time, grow tired of repeated injections. Some men can't conceive of sticking a needle into their penises. In the United States, only 60 percent of patients continue past the first year and 25 percent after two years—far fewer than their European counterparts. It's our feeling that if after six to twelve months their condition doesn't revert to "normal," many men will opt for the permanent solution—a penile implant.

Who should use PEP? PEP is an excellent alternative for people with potentially reversible impotence—for example, men with spinal cord injuries or psychogenic impotence. And it may prove satisfactory for the many men who are not certain that their impotence is permanent.

Who should not use PEP? PEP, however, is not medically recommended for everyone. Papaverine and Regitine may interact with other drugs, such as with central nervous system depressants and morphine-based pain medications. And there is a concern that PEP might cause liver disease. Men taking these drugs should have frequent liver function tests performed. Patients with severe cardiovascular problems—especially cardiac arrhythmias—should not use PEP. In addition, papaverine interferes with the therapeutic effects of levodopa in patients with Parkinson's disease. Conditions that may preclude using PEP therapy include:

Alcoholism
Cardiac arrhythmias, cardiac problems
Consumption of central nervous system depressants and morphine-based pain medications
Hepatitis
Liver disease
Obese men who cannot see their penis
Parkinson's patients taking L-dopa
Postpriapism impotence
Severe venous leakage
Sickle-cell anemia

What are the potential side effects of PEP? Minor side effects include local reactions such as bleeding, bruising, swelling, and discomfort at the injection site. Local injury to the urethra and infection are also potential problems. Continued injections may cause scarring (fibrosis) of the underlying tissue. PEP may cause liver disease, especially for men with liver problems, alcoholism, or hepatitis.

In addition, PEP may create a prolonged erection (priapismlike) requiring immediate medical intervention to avoid damage to the internal penile structures. Usually an injection of epinephrine will counteract the drug and allow the penis to become flaccid. Occasionally, however, the physician must aspirate a small amount of blood or shunt it out of the penis to reduce the pressure. If treated quickly, this will not cause permanent damage. However, prolonged erections can cause permanent organic impotence—something a psychogenically impotent man should consider. If the drug is administered according to the physician's instructions, the risk of experiencing a priapismlike erection is very small.

The long-term effects of using PEP are unknown. Few controlled scientific studies have been performed.

Prostaglandin E_1 Injection Therapy

A Japanese report presented at the International Society for Impotence Research in Prague in 1986 showed that prostaglandin E_1 (PGE_1) is effective in producing good-quality erections when it is injected directly into the penis. A powerful smooth-muscle relaxant like papaverine/Regitine, PGE_1 (Prostin VR) produces fewer side effects such as prolonged erection and deleterious effects on liver function. As it has a nearly neutral pH, the solution is also less caustic to penile tissues. (Though FDA-approved in connection with infant heart conditions, PGE_1 has not yet been approved for treating impotence.) The main disadvantage is that it costs about three times as much as papaverine/Regitine injections do.

EXTERNAL MANAGEMENT DEVICES

A number of men who object to injection therapy, or who are not ready to seek a more permanent solution such as an implant, choose to use an external management device. This type of treatment is noninvasive and reversible in that it can be discontinued at any time. These devices utilize, in varying degrees, one or both principles of vacuum and entrapment. The latter creates a pressure around the base of the penis by means of a flexible ring or band to keep the blood from leaving the penis. The vacuum is made possible by means of a tube or shaped cover being placed over the entire penis and a vacuum created.

When using a vacuum-and-entrapment-type device, the penis normally becomes firm; however, it does not become "erect" because it may lack stability. You may notice a slight wobble. However, most patients are satisfied with the quality of the erection and are able to have satisfactory penile-vaginal intercourse.

Unfortunately, these devices, requiring preparation, do not permit total spontaneity in lovemaking. And some men report that the entrapment ring placed around the base of the penis causes discomfort during ejaculation because the ejaculate becomes trapped in the urethra. This problem may be relieved by loosening or removing the entrapment ring prior to ejaculation. *Constriction for more than thirty minutes is considered unsafe.*

Many couples report good results. One woman approached us at a medical convention and told us that she and her husband had had poor-quality sex for the first twenty years of their marriage and nonexistent sex for the last ten. Then their urologist recommended that they use an external management device, and they were both happy with the results. Another man told us he wouldn't take $1,000 for his entrapment system.

Who should not use external management devices? Patients with sickle-cell anemia, or those who are taking anticoagulant therapy, have a higher risk of priapism and should not use vacuum devices.

Types of External Management Devices

Mechanical management devices fall into the following two major categories: vacuum and nonvacuum. All of these devices will enable the man and his partner to achieve successful penile-vaginal intercourse. *When used as recommended, FDA-approved devices are safe* and will cause no damage to delicate penile structures. In addition, each device comes with instructions on how to use it when pregnancy is desired.

VACUUM DEVICES

With entrapment. These devices pull a gentle vacuum over the penis, causing it to engorge with blood. After sufficient rigidity is attained, an entrapment ring is slipped around the base of the penis, trapping the blood and sustaining the erection throughout intercourse.

The device works by inserting the penis, with the base well lubricated, into a plastic cylinder and then creating a controlled vacuum by means of a hand pump. After the penis is engorged, the user places an entrapment ring at the base of the penis. The penis will remain rigid until the ring is removed.

Nonentrapment. These devices employ a vacuum that gently draws the well-lubricated penis into a pressure-sensitive clear silicone sheath (resembling a condom). The vacuum created by sucking on a tube connected to the device causes blood to engorge the penis, thus creating an erection. A soft, nonconstrictive collar placed around the base of the penis allows additional arterial blood to enter the penis but prevents venous leakage.

NONVACUUM DEVICES

With entrapment. These devices are particularly useful for men who can attain an erection but, due to venous leakage, lose it before lovemaking is complete. Once the man achieves a firm, "natural" erection, he slips an entrapment ring around the base of his penis, trapping the blood and maintaining the erection until the ring is removed. (Men who have difficulty achieving a firm erection can improve the blood flow into the penis by gently massaging the main artery leading to the penis—stroking the artery from the rectum to the base of the penis.)

Nonentrapment. These structural support devices physically support the flaccid penis and can provide—without engorgement—sufficient penile support for penetration.

When using any of these external management devices, it's very important to *follow the manufacturer's instructions* and not leave entrapment rings on beyond the recommended time limit. Failure to do so could cause severe damage. When the instructions are followed carefully, external management devices can be safe and effective to use.

ELECTROSTIMULATORY DEVICE

Rather new on the horizon is a device that creates an erection by electrically stimulating the nerves and blood vessels serving the penis. This self-contained, battery-operated device is inserted into the anus and controlled remotely by the user. The electrical current is quite low, and users report no pain or discomfort. Urologists can test the effectiveness of the device in the office. In fact, some urologists employ the Male Electronic Genital Stimulator (MEGS) for diagnosing impotence.

This electrostimulatory device is well suited for men with nerve disease or with psychogenic impotence. The vascular system must be intact for the device to work. (At the time this book was being written, electrostimulatory devices were in the experimental, clinical-trial stage and not available for general use.)

INTERNAL DEVICES (PENILE IMPLANTS)

Penile implants are said to be the most "natural" method for overcoming the effects of chronic impotence. Completely concealed inside the body, penile implants come in a number of different configurations, which are described in some detail below. All implants require the surgical implantation of two rods or cylinders into the shaft of the penis. And all implant components are made of or encased in silicone plastic, which is compatible with the body. The type of penile implant you select should be compatible with your body build, genital anatomy, physical dexterity, expectations, emotional needs, and financial resources. The selection requires cooperation and advice from the sexual partner as well as from the urologist.

What Are the Different Types of Penile Implants?

SEMIRIGID

The semirigid device consists of two semirigid plastic rods that are surgically implanted into the two areas of the penis, the corpora cavernosa. The rods are stiff enough to permit penetration and flexible enough to permit placement of the penis on the thigh or abdomen for cosmetic purposes. Although the shaft of the penis is rigid, the head of the penis (glans) does not swell during intercourse. (Because of this, some people use an external management device along with an implant. You should check with your urologist before doing this, though.) In either case, partners report that the semirigid implant is very satisfactory. Generally, this is the least expensive implant and requires less extensive surgery (and a shorter hospital stay) than fully inflatable implants. Semirigid devices are particularly attractive to men with limited dexterity, such as men who have Parkinson's disease, or muscular paralysis following brain surgery for a tumor.

HINGED

The hinged device is made of a solid flexible rod that has a hingelike action at the base of the penis so it can be placed in the upright or flaccid position. The rods are surgically implanted into the corpora cavernosa of the penis. The "hinge" makes it easier to bend out of place for cosmetic purposes. The hinged device is relatively inexpensive and requires less extensive surgery than fully inflatable implants.

MALLEABLE

The malleable implant has a flexible core that "remembers" the position it is placed in. Once bent, the malleable implant tends to remain in that position: upright for lovemaking and downward, close to the body, for other activities. Although a bit more expensive than the semirigid implant, the malleable device offers cosmetic advantages. Three months after his radical prostate cancer surgery, Neil had a malleable device implanted with very good results.

SELF-CONTAINED

Self-contained penile implants come in two versions: nonfluid mechanical and fluid.

Nonfluid mechanical. This silicone-covered device contains a series of cuplike units operated by wire and springs. Gently bending the penis at midshaft creates pressure on the wire, which changes the state from flaccidity to rigidity, and vice versa.

Fluid. This implant contains a reservoir filled with fluid (usually saline) within each of two cylinders placed in the shaft of the penis. The cylinders can be filled by gently pressing them near the glans of the penis. Pressing the release valve between the middle of the penis and the glans, or (with some models) bending the penis at midshaft, allows the fluid to flow back into the reservoir for a flaccid state. Although these devices fill, they do not inflate, so the erection is not quite as full as with a fully inflatable device.

Self-contained fluid inflatable devices gain their popularity because of simplicity and because they require a less extensive surgical procedure than fully inflatable implants.

FULLY INFLATABLE

A simple hydraulic system, the multicomponent, fully inflatable penile implant contains a fluid reservoir that is surgically placed within the abdomen, two inflatable penile cylinders placed in the shaft of the penis, and a pump-and-deflate mechanism placed in the scrotum. Tubing connects the three components to allow for the transfer of fluid. In some models the reservoir is combined with the pump-and-deflate mechanism concealed in the scrotum. The degree of erection can be varied by manipulating the pump. And the erection will appear and feel natural. The degree of flaccidity can also be controlled with the release mechanism. The surgery, however, is more involved and usually requires a longer recovery. In addition, the fully inflatable device is the most expensive one to have implanted.

How Is the Surgery Done?

First, this type of surgery should only be performed by a urologist specialist with extensive experience in this type of surgery. The type of *incision* is based on the patient's history of previous surgeries as well as the physician's experiences and preferences.

Many physicians use the peno-scrotal incision, which is a 2-centimeter (1.5 inch) incision that follows along the midline underneath the penis from the base of the penis toward the scrotum. The peno-scrotal incision causes the least complications and, for the multicomponent inflatable device, requires the shortest tubing. This reduces potential kinking problems.

Some physicians still prefer to use the original, suprapubic incision, which is placed horizontally (sometimes vertically) above the pubic bone.

The nonfluid mechanical devices can also be inserted into the corpora cavernosa through two small (penile) incisions placed near the tip of the penis, near where the foreskin joins.

In contrast to the fully inflatable devices, the self-contained, malleable, hinged, or semirigid devices require less invasive surgery because they are implanted into the shaft of the penis, between the thick envelope of the corpora and the spongy tissue that normally fills with blood during engorgement.

Most patients report to the hospital the morning of surgery. The actual operation requires anywhere from one-half hour to two hours, depending on the type of device selected. Hospital stays range from two to four days, with surgeries for self-contained and semirigid implants requiring much shorter stays than those for multicomponent devices. Usually an antibiotic is given to avoid a staph infection—a complication that affects only 1 to 2 percent of patients. (Some physicians are beginning to implant the self-contained semirigid devices on an outpatient basis.)

Does It Hurt?

The reaction to any type of surgery is very individual. Most men report that they experience pain for two to three days following the surgery. Depending on their tolerance to pain, some men require medication; others do not. Local sensitivity or discomfort may continue for up to two weeks, or more for some. Healing continues for the first six weeks, much as with any type of surgery. See the list of tips for surgical recovery.

Tips for Surgical Recovery

Wear comfortable clothing—for example, a loose night shirt.

Some men report they are most comfortable with their genitalia hanging free; however, others report relief with gentle support from jockey shorts or an athletic supporter. If you receive a fully inflatable implant, let the genitalia hang free so the pump mechanism remains properly placed.

Lie on your side with a pillow placed between your knees and rest your genitalia on the inside of your thigh.

Use a heating pad or hot water bottle where it hurts.

Soak in a warm tub of water—it's heavenly! *Caution:* Check with your doctor first, however, because your incision must be completely healed before you get it wet. This takes about a week.

Avoid becoming constipated.

Ask your doctor for pain medication if you need it.

Take your antibiotics as recommended by your urologist.

Leave your inflatable device alone until you receive instructions from your urologist.

Avoid sexual intercourse for four to six weeks.

Do what's comfortable; if it hurts, don't do it.

Total bed rest is not needed; walking is fine, but treat yourself tenderly.

When Can I Go Back to Work?

You will probably want to plan for two weeks of rest before you gradually get back into the swing of things. Most men can return to an office job in a week or so, or to a job requiring heavy lifting in three weeks. Discuss this with your doctor.

We Suggest . . .

No matter what method you select, you may find that a lubricant will help you with penile-vaginal intercourse. If at first the woman is tense, she may not lubricate well, much as when you first had sex. This extra help may ease you both.

Making the "right" choice is strictly a decision between you, your urologist, and your partner. All of the methods described in this chapter work well. Some men still in the twilight zone of indecision may prefer a less permanent treatment, such as penile injections. Some men who don't want to spend substantial sums for surgery may prefer an external management device. And others who want to simulate nature more permanently may opt for an implant.

Choice of treatment may be expanded in the future. At the time of this book's publication progress is being made toward: patches similar to those used in the nitroglycerin transdermal infusion system; pills and powders that can be taken orally; and further development in the treatment of *venogenic* (venous leakage) impotence.

In this chapter we've tried to familiarize you with the options you have so that you can investigate them further with regard to your unique situation and acceptances at a given point in time. The "right" choice is your decision to make, subject, of course, to any medical considerations.

8

WHEN IT *IS* IN YOUR HEAD

You have up to a 1 in 5 chance that the origin of your impotence is purely "all in your head" (psychological). This is a dramatically lower figure than you might have heard in the late 1970s, when the medical community felt that 90 percent of impotence was "in your head."

Today health experts advise us that psychological factors are the primary cause of chronic impotence (*inhibited sexual excitement*) in 20 to 25 percent of cases and are *complicating factors* in nearly 100 percent of *all* impotence. This *psychological overlay,* affecting nearly all impotent men and their partners, frequently responds to counseling, sex therapy, or marriage counseling.

Psychotherapy and similar approaches can be very helpful for the man experiencing chronic psychogenic impotence; but when used indiscriminately, it can actually *harm* the organically impotent man by overlooking his potentially serious medical condition. As we have stated before, it's very important that you receive an accurate medical diagnosis before you seek help from a mental-health professional.

DIAGNOSING CHRONIC PSYCHOGENIC IMPOTENCE

No psychological test can determine if your impotence is purely psychogenic in origin. The only way accurately to diagnose chronic psychogenic impotence is to eliminate organic impotence as the cause. If you have an erectile problem that persists for five weeks or more, you need to consult with a urologist specialist for a medical evaluation. Don't try to play doctor, as we did. Only a qualified urologist can determine whether physical factors or psychological factors are the source of your erectile problem (see Chapter 4, "Evaluating Impotence"). As many psychiatrists have advised us, "Don't assume it's all in your head until your urologist tells you it is."

As a rule of thumb, and in contrast to organic impotence, the onset of psychogenic impotence is generally acute and sudden. This sudden onset may be associated with some emotionally traumatic event, such as the death of a spouse or rejection from a lover.

Tom was devastated when, two weeks before their wedding, his fiancée eloped with his best friend. It was over a year before he even asked another woman out for a date. When their relationship began to warm up, he found that with sexual arousal also came the memories of his fiancée's desertion. Within seconds he'd lose all amorous emotions *and* his erection. With counseling, Tom overcame his problem.

The psychogenically impotent man may report that he has good-quality, spontaneous erections at times when he does not plan to have intercourse. And he may obtain good erections with masturbation or with partners other than his usual partner. These experiences suggest that the source of his impotence is not due to physical impairment.

Chronic psychogenic impotence should not be confused with temporary (situational) impotence, which virtually all men experience at one time or another; or with intermittent or partial impotence, which many organically impotent men experience.

If the urologist specialist can find no physical reason for your impotence, you need to consult with a mental-health professional who is familiar with treating impotent men. Working with your urologist, the mental-health professional can outline a treatment plan best suited to your particular situation. In addition to counseling, this plan may include short-term medical treatment, such as injection therapy or the use of external management devices—or in particularly resistant cases, long-term medical resolution with a penile implant. Depending on the nature of the problem, the therapist also may recommend counseling for the partner.

You can find a qualified therapist by asking your urologist, by attending an I.A. or I-Anon meeting, or by writing to I.A. and requesting a referral.

COMMON CAUSES OF PSYCHOGENIC IMPOTENCE

Performance Anxiety

Probably the most common cause of psychogenic impotence is performance anxiety or the fear of failure. This condition often begins when the man loses his erection before or during coitus because of some kind of stress, anxiety, or distraction. Embarrassed and anxious, during his next attempt at lovemaking the man may become preoccupied with thoughts about his previous failure. His heightened anxiety interferes even further with his sexual enjoyment and causes another failure. If this happens several times, his self-consciousness may increase to the point that he believes he is completely impotent and will never be able to have successful sexual relations again.

Ralph reported to us that when his wife was out of town, he attempted to masturbate and failed to get an erection. From that point on, he had trouble getting erections. Panicked, he consulted a sex therapist. In his mind he had built a temporary problem into a chronic impotence situation. When the counselor helped restore his self-confidence, his psychogenic impotence was reversed.

Please recognize that this same sequence of events can occur during the early stages of an organic problem. And the psychological overlay—anxiety about your performance—will appear exactly the same. You cannot merely assume that because you are anxious about your performance, you are psychogenically impotent. If your condition persists for five weeks, you need to consult with a urologist specialist to determine the true source of the problem.

Sometimes performance anxiety resolves itself—an understanding partner helps relieve the man's stress, or a few successful experiences restore his self-confidence. Chapter 9, "Treatments for Psychogenic Impotence," will explain the counseling techniques used to help overcome performance anxiety.

Inability to Meet Cultural Expectations

In a society filled with pressures to be physically fit, to look like a lifeguard, and to be a financial success, it's little wonder that some men experience a problem with their self-image. Traditionally, the man has been portrayed as the breadwinner, protector, and dominant sexual partner. Magazines, television, and movies have extended and reinforced this fantasy by depicting an unrealistic image of what a "real" man should be.

Certainly most men will never live up to such macho

stereotypes as John Wayne, James Bond, Mike Hammer, and Prince Charming. Nor can men expect to achieve the unrealistic levels of arousal or performance suggested in sexually explicit photographs and movies. And yet many men are disappointed in themselves if they cannot.

Such disappointments may lead to anxiety and depression, both of which can reduce sexual desire and adversely affect performance in the bedroom.

Premature Ejaculation

Premature ejaculation refers to a condition where the man—on an intermittent or regular basis—cannot prevent ejaculation before his partner has been sexually satisfied. Following ejaculation, his penis becomes flaccid until his normal physical recovery (*refractory*) period has passed. By then, however, the mood may have changed, the man feels inadequate, and both partners are left dissatisfied. Premature ejaculation is not the same as impotence. However, because the man cannot gain and maintain his erection long enough for his partner to be satisfied, we want to address this condition briefly.

Premature ejaculation is almost always a psychogenic problem. As such it responds well to psychiatric treatment that focuses on finding stressful factors in the relationship. Sensate focus exercises can improve the couple's communication and extend their periods of pleasurable intimacy, short of intercourse. Also, during foreplay, the woman can squeeze the man's penis firmly to avert ejaculation. Repeated exercises of this sort will help the couple achieve longer and longer periods of "endurance" in sexual intercourse before ejaculation.

Lack of Self-Esteem

Sometimes a failed relationship can have a very destructive effect on self-esteem. After his fiancée broke off their engagement, John believed that no one would be interested in him, and he feared initiating another relationship. John didn't want to develop close emotional attachments that would increase his chances of being hurt again. His psychogenic impotence provided a perfect excuse for not pursuing a new relationship.

Men with inadequate self-esteem often feel unworthy of having a sexual relationship with a woman. They may believe, as Phil did, that their performance is unsatisfactory in spite of the fact that it generally has been okay. Psychogenic impotence protects these men from forming close sexual relationships.

Marital Discord

Marital discord is an extremely common cause of psychogenic impotence. An angry husband may consciously or unconsciously withdraw or refrain from sex as a way of punishing or avoiding his wife.

Joe's psychogenic impotence resulted from years of coping with an alcoholic wife. His inability to perform provided the perfect excuse for not trying. Bill became impotent as a result of recurring financial worries that, over time, had destroyed his marital relationship. Sam was simply bored with a wife who mistakenly thought her purely passive sexual role was what her husband wanted. Not only did Sam's impotence give him an excuse not to have sex with his wife, but it also served to keep him faithful.

Psychogenic impotence often arises from poor sexual communication with the partner. As Gene became older, he found that to gain an erection, he needed more manual stimulation during foreplay. Because "talking about sex" was always a taboo, he was unable to tell his partner what he needed. Accompanied by a high level of frustration, their attempts at lovemaking often failed.

Sometimes a change in marital roles affects a couple's relationship. Bob began experiencing erectile problems when his wife went to work after he was injured in an accident. No longer able to provide for his family, Bob didn't feel like a complete man any more. These emotions spilled over into their sexual relationship when he became unable to achieve an erection.

Professional counseling and the restoration of good communication often overcome marital discord and lead to the resumption of a satisfactory sexual relationship. Chapter 9 will tell more about how counseling can help.

Widowhood

Occasionally the death of a spouse can bring on psychogenic impotence. Herman reported to an I.A. group that his problems with impotence showed up a year after his wife's death. At that time he started seeing a woman he and his deceased wife had known for over twenty years. After a few months he developed amorous feelings for this woman. When he attempted to act upon these feelings, however, he was unable to get an erection. He told the I.A. members that he attributed the problem to his recent prostate surgery.

The men at the I.A. meeting encouraged Herman to see a urologist specialist as soon as possible. A complete medical evaluation revealed that no physical problem caused Herman's impotence. After several weeks in counseling, Herman realized that his problem stemmed from the guilt he harbored over his betrayal of his lost partner. Herman soon overcame his guilt feelings and, the last we heard, he and his new partner were planning a honeymoon in the Caribbean.

Religious Inhibitions

Most religions discourage sexual intercourse outside of marriage. In an attempt to discourage premarital sex, some parents go so far as to teach youngsters that sex is dirty. Sometimes the feelings of guilt about sex are instilled so strongly that they become anxiety provoking even in marriage.

Matthew had a very moralistic and rigid upbringing. When he married Heather, he couldn't escape feeling that there was something sinful about his sexual desires. Because sex wasn't something "nice" people talk about—particularly with a lady—it was difficult for either of them to understand each other's feelings. They couldn't discuss what was pleasurable, uncomfortable, painful, or distasteful. After two years Matthew still was unable to consummate their marriage. At that time Heather insisted that he see a doctor, because in the eyes of their church, their marriage could not be recognized unless it was consummated. When the doctor could find no physical reason for Matthew's impotence, he referred them for marriage counseling.

Matthew and Heather learned from their marriage counselor that *poor communication* is the largest single source of sexual difficulties. The primary focus of their treatment centered around improving their communication. In time, Matthew was able to overcome his anxiety and develop a normal sexual relationship with his wife.

The fear of inducing pregnancy is another source of anxiety for many men who have been brought up to believe that sexual intercourse is only meant for procreation, not recreation, that contraception is sinful. The fear of having children, or of having too large a family to care for, may cause the man to suppress his feelings, curb his interest, and develop an erection problem.

Guilt

Feelings of guilt can be very disruptive to a sexual relationship. Guilt may stem from a number of sources, including an extramarital affair, homosexual fantasies, or the loss of a spouse through death.

Harry felt so guilty about having an illicit affair that he couldn't face making love with his spouse. Psychogenic impotence provided the perfect excuse for avoiding his conflict. It was only after receiving counseling that Harry was able to resolve his problem.

Curious about recurring homosexual fantasies, one day Mark went to a homosexual bar and decided to experiment. Terrorized by this single episode, he thought that he was exclusively homosexual and unable to have a future with a woman. When he did fall in love with a woman, his anxiety about homosexuality made him impotent and prevented him from developing a sexual relationship. After suffering through three failed relationships, Mark consulted a therapist. The therapist referred him for a urological workup, which proved to be negative. After that, the therapist could effectively deal with Mark's psychological problems.

Sexual Abuse

With surprising frequency, male children are the subjects of sexual abuse and exploitation by older children and adults. This varies in severity and frequency, and in the child's and family's reactions to the situation. Often when the abused child reaches adulthood, he remains deeply affected by these early experiences. Poor self-esteem and sexual maladjustment often are the results.

Having learned during childhood to associate sexual experiences with deep feelings of anger and guilt, the victim may find that these painful emotions reawaken during sexual encounters. These strong feelings may interfere with intimacy and with developing a mutually satisfying sexual relationship. Counseling is usually needed to resolve these feelings and to build self-esteem.

Then the individual can learn to experience his sexuality in a pleasurable fashion, without reliving his early childhood experiences.

Masturbation

Many religions frown upon masturbation, in spite of the known fact that almost every youngster and adult has practiced it—many on a fairly regular basis. Often boys are told that if they masturbate, they will go blind or their penis will fall off.

When faced with declining erectile ability, some men feel that masturbating has worn out their penis, or that their impotence is the punishment wrought for their sexual "transgressions."

We know that masturbation has no detrimental effect on sexual function. In fact, regular sexual activity of any type tends to increase sexual interest and appetite by maintaining higher levels of testosterone circulating.

Men anxious about this problem should seek counseling.

Depression

A lack of sexual desire, or loss of libido, is one of the primary symptoms of depression. Other symptoms include sadness, lack of energy, lack of pleasure in previously enjoyable activities, loss of appetite, insomnia, and in extreme cases, thoughts of suicide.

Less severe forms of depression may simply be described as feeling blue, lacking energy, or experiencing increased irritability. When some men become depressed, they become so preoccupied with their health and physical symptoms and often develop unfounded beliefs that they are unable to perform sexually, or are undesirable sexual partners.

Depression can be triggered by a number of personal

losses or failures, including the loss of a job, falling short of goals, making poor grades, missing a promotion, marital problems, financial problems, and suffering a business failure. Depression may also be brought on by prolonged sickness and persistent pain, or by taking certain medications.

Robert became so dissatisfied with his marriage that he buried himself in his work. When he did come home he was exhausted and unable to participate in family activities or in any form of play. He'd lost track of all of his friends and felt trapped in an unhappy marriage and life-style. Plagued by a series of business disappointments, Robert became even more despondent. His depression and strenuous life-style finally took its toll, first causing impotence, and later a heart attack. Having ignored an early symptom of arteriosclerosis—impotence—Robert and his wife now found themselves coping with a potentially life-threatening health problem.

It was difficult for them to know if Robert's depression, life-style, or blood-vessel disease was the primary culprit. But in the final analysis, it didn't matter which came first. When Robert received appropriate medical treatment and he and his wife received marriage counseling, they were able to rekindle the emotional fires they once enjoyed.

Secondary Gain

A man may become psychogenically impotent to avoid a distasteful or anxiety-provoking situation, or to gain some perceived reward.

When Henry's wife left him, his male ego was crushed. Feeling sorry for himself, he assumed the role of a martyr. He gained a great deal of sympathy from his family and friends. After a year of "mourning," Henry met a woman for whom he cared a great deal.

When he ended up in the bedroom with her, however, his subconscious mind decided that he couldn't justify his role as martyr and be a successful lover too. He wasn't ready to give up the benefits he'd gained from his martyrdom, so his mind made sure that his body could not perform. Actually this also worked out to Henry's benefit because with his sexual failure, his partner lavished even more sympathy and support on him. But Henry needed to learn to enjoy the present instead of living in the past.

Please keep in mind that, in retrospect, it often seems easy to explain why a man develops psychogenic impotence. However, psychogenic impotence is not something a man chooses consciously to punish himself or a loved one. Psychogenic impotence is just as real to its victim as organic impotence is.

PSYCHOLOGICAL FACTORS COMPLICATING ORGANIC IMPOTENCE

A man with an organic impotence problem more often than not develops psychological problems (overlays) that complicate his physical problem. Having experienced a few erection failures resulting from a temporary physical problem, David became embarrassed and scared. Fearing future failures, his anxiety contributed to his physical problem and led to more failures. What started out as a borderline physical problem, aggravated by ingesting alcohol and nicotine, became a chronic impotence problem caused by a combination of physical and psychological factors.

If David had sought an accurate urological diagnosis when his problem first developed, he and his partner could have avoided years of heartache and anxiety.

It's almost the exception for an organically impotent man and his partner not to experience emotional problems. Virtually every couple dealing with an impotence problem could benefit from counseling.

In the next chapter you will learn about the treatment options available for psychogenically impotent men and for organically impotent men who also have psychological overlays.

9

TREATMENTS FOR PSYCHOGENIC IMPOTENCE

Nearly every couple who has experienced impotence—for whatever cause—can benefit from counseling. When we speak at conventions and to I.A. groups, we tell people that 20 percent of impotence is purely physical, 20 percent is purely psychological, and the 60 percent remaining is a combination, in varying proportions, of both physical and psychological problems. In nearly every case of chronic impotence, both the impotent man and the partner experience associated emotional problems.

Even if you (or your partner) have been diagnosed as having a physical cause for the impotence, we encourage you to read this chapter. The information discussed may give you some insights into how counseling also can help you and your partner adjust.

IS COUNSELING FOR YOU?

First of all, you should get a complete medical evaluation from a urologist specializing in impotence before you seek counseling. Sometimes the reassurance from test results that reveal you are physically capable of having an erection helps a lot. Only after you know the cause of your impotence—physical or emotional—can counseling be beneficial.

Counseling and psychotherapy may be useful in the following situations:

Psychogenic impotence without physical causes. Long-standing psychogenic impotence may indicate the existence of deeply rooted emotional problems extending back to one's childhood. In addition, chronic impotence of any kind may cause serious damage to the partner relationship. Often counseling for the impotent man and for the partner can help the couple return to a healthy sexual relationship.

Combination of psychogenic and physical impotence. Physical illness almost always causes an emotional response. But when that illness is related to one's sexuality, it can be devastating. Counseling for these couples will promote the most effective response to medical and surgical treatment and enhance the return to normal sexual relations.

Nicotine, alcohol, or drug abuse. Sometimes when the use of these substances is brought under control, partial or complete potency will return. For example, by stopping cigarette smoking, a man may improve blood-flow problems associated with blood-vessel constriction. Or by stopping marijuana smoking, a man can improve his testosterone level. Where applicable, a physician will recommend that an addiction be controlled prior to recommending medical intervention. A number of excellent treatment programs and support groups such as Alcoholics Anonymous and AL-Anon are available to help a couple with these problems. After the alcohol or drug dependence is brought under control, counseling for the impotence problem or relationship problem may prove beneficial.

UNDERSTANDING THE PROBLEM

The therapist will first try to identify the basis for the impotence problem and for the relationship problem with the partner. Then he or she will determine the best method for resolving the anger, guilt, anxiety, inhibitions, and other factors involved in the impotence situation.

Sometimes the causes for the psychogenic impotence and for the relationship problem are the same, as in Lester and Valerie's case. Through a series of interviews, the therapist learned that this couple had had a good sexual relationship for more than two years. When Valerie became dissatisfied with Lester's reluctance to tie the knot permanently, she started pushing him about getting married. At one point she even threatened to break off their relationship if he didn't agree. Distressed by her threats, Lester experienced his first erection failure. Taking full advantage of his "impotence" episode, Valerie started giving him an even harder time—questioning his manhood and blaming him for her unhappiness. Ridden with anger and lowered self-esteem, Lester became completely impotent. The therapist told Lester and Valerie that they had several problems to work on. Lester needed to find out why he was reluctant to make a long-term commitment to Valerie. And they both needed to learn how to communicate their feelings and to "fight fair" without destroying one another's egos.

Sometimes the causes for the psychogenic impotence and for the relationship problem are quite different, as in Lee and Audrey's situation. Lee told the therapist that he had grown up believing that sex was a "wham, bam, thank you ma'am" affair. Though usually left sexually dissatisfied, his wife told the therapist that she accepted Lee's behavior as "normal." Because Audrey saw Lee as the master of the household, she didn't dare criticize his performance in the bedroom.

Eventually Lee became bored with his wife's passive approach to lovemaking and decided to experiment with an attractive secretary at the office. Ridden with anxiety and guilt, he was unable to perform with the secretary and, subsequently, with Audrey.

Fortunately, after six miserable months, Audrey saw us on a national television program and mustered up enough courage to go to an I-Anon meeting held in her local community. When she learned that help was available, she encouraged Lee to go to an I.A. meeting.

After consulting with a urologist and receiving a thorough medical evaluation, they decided to seek marriage counseling. In addition to recommending counseling for both of them, the therapist recommended sensate focus exercises to help them improve their sexual communication.

As with the urologist specialist, it is crucial that you do not withhold information from the therapist. Only when all of the facts are on the table, so to speak, can the therapist outline necessary treatment. A competent therapist will respect your wishes for confidentiality and will not disclose embarrassing or damaging information to a partner.

COUNSELING TECHNIQUES

Importance of Good Communication

A major goal of psychotherapy is to facilitate good communication about sexual and nonsexual matters. The couple needs to learn how to express positive and negative feelings, and they need to increase their sensitivity to each other's needs—particularly in the bedroom. When both partners feel free to communicate their needs and desires, their sense of shame at making certain requests or their fear of hurting their partner's feelings by giving directives or constructive criticism is reduced.

Communication also must be reestablished on a physical, nonverbal level. This may be accomplished by means of sensual or sexual homework exercises. (Single people without partners may benefit from the services of a sex surrogate.) Enhanced communication allows partners to get to know each other on a completely new level.

Sensate Focus Exercises

Sensate focus exercises were introduced many years ago by William Masters and Virginia Johnson. These therapeutic exercises were developed to improve sexual function. They make individuals more aware of the sexual aspects of their bodies. The therapist instructs the couple to explore each other's body and erogenous zones in the privacy of their own home. At first, they are told to please each other without any direct genital manipulation. The reactions to these exercises are discussed with the therapist during succeeding sessions. The therapist progressively alters the instructions to allow increasing levels of genital stimulation culminating, after several weeks, in sexual intercourse.

Sensate focusing is a powerful technique for overcoming performance anxiety and lack of sexual communication and awareness on the part of either or both partners.

Medical Support

Occasionally psychogenic impotence is slow to respond to psychotherapy. In these situations, the therapist will work with the urologist to find a temporary medical solution to the impotence problem. After several weeks of counseling, Matt reported to his therapist that when he was having intercourse, rather than being able to enjoy what was happening, his mind was always thinking about his next step. Coupled with his unrealistic performance expectations, this led to repeated failures. The therapist thought Matt was trying too hard. Hoping to increase Matt's confidence, the therapist recommended that Matt use injection therapy or an external management device until things improved. With his performance anxiety under control, Matt soon found that he no longer needed medical support.

Sometimes the psychogenic impotence is so deeply rooted that the man decides prolonged therapy is not the answer. Hugh revealed to us he was terrified of making his partner pregnant, so he avoided all emotional attachments. He viewed childbirth as a painful and agonizing thing to put his loved one through, so unconsciously he began to avoid all emotional attachments by becoming psychogenically impotent.

After a couple of years of psychotherapy, Hugh fell deeply in love with a very nice woman. But even though he had a strong physical attraction to her, he still was unable to get an erection. He wanted to marry her but didn't think it was fair to her to marry while he was still impotent. So he decided to get an implant. He told us afterward that he and his partner were extremely satisfied with their newfound sexuality. Several months later we received a wedding announcement.

COUNSELING FOR PSYCHOLOGICAL OVERLAYS

Before medical treatment can effectively restore sexuality, psychological factors must be resolved. Counseling may assist the couple greatly by helping them prioritize the treatment of complex emotional and physical disorders that are both frightening and embarrassing to them. Also, counseling will allow the partners to explore their expectations and to compare them with treatment results obtained by others. In addition, the therapist can educate the couple by answering questions and concerns about the disorder and treatment.

Many men and women report that they can achieve these goals by attending I.A. and I-Anon meetings. Dennis and Charlene told us that they benefited greatly by being able to talk with people who had experienced what they were going through and by having access to medical advisors willing to share their experience and know-how.

As Bruce tells I.A. chapter members, "Fixing your penis is only the first step. After that's done, you need to work at rebuilding your relationship." Chapter 10, "Starting Your New Life Together," will tell how, once you have overcome your impotence, you can get on with the rest of your life.

10

STARTING YOUR NEW LIFE TOGETHER

"I'm not sure I want to return to a *normal* sex life," Vivien said as she puffed nervously on her fourth cigarette. "He hasn't been the most *pleasant* man to live with these past twelve years."

Several other women at the I-Anon meeting laughed. But they didn't laugh *at* Vivien. They laughed because they too had had similar thoughts.

"I know what you mean," Jessica said. "I've been walking on eggshells so long, I don't think I know what *is* normal anymore."

"Yeah," Janet agreed. "Our relationship has cooled off so much, I'm not sure where to start. I can't even remember the last time we held hands—let alone made love."

"There's more to getting back to a normal life than getting his penis fixed," Eileen MacKenzie cautioned. "And most of us need some help along the way."

"She's right," Joan said. "When Walter decided to get an implant, I had a million questions. What should I do? What should I *not* do? Will it hurt me? Will I be able to tell the difference? Am *I* turning him on?—At first, I didn't know who to turn to . . ."

While the I-Anon conversation continued, in the next room at the I.A. meeting their impotent partners were sharing their concerns.

"I know this may sound unreasonable," Louis said, "but I thought that my implant would make everything okay again. But it hasn't."

"Don't feel alone," Mel said. "It took Blanche and me months just to become friends again."

Dick laughed. "Yeah, you can't just turn back the clock—like nothing ever happened."

"You can say that again," Eric said. "When I go on a date, I never know if I should *tell* or *not tell.*"

"What difference does it make?" Bruce MacKenzie asked. "The important thing is the relationship that you have with your partner—the caring, the communication, the warmth and affection—not what is making your penis stiff."

The I.A. group laughed.

"Bruce, you always have a way of cutting through the garbage," Eric said. "We're still uptight about getting it up, when we should be concerned about getting our lives back together."

Couples who seek early treatment—before the psychogenic overlay becomes an integral part of their daily lives—and couples who maintain good communication have fewer problems adjusting to their *renewed* sexual relationship. Unfortunately, though, by the time most impotent men and their partners get medical help, they have already endured year after year of watching their relationship crumble.

Getting the penis fixed is only the *first step* in the long road to recovery and discovery—to starting your new life together. As Eileen told the I-Anon group, "After long periods of celibacy, resumption of sexual relations is very much like trying to ride a bicycle again. You may never forget, but you're a little wobbly at first." We find that most couples can benefit from professional counseling and from attending support groups such as I.A. for impotent men and I-Anon for partners.

WHAT'S "NORMAL"?

After months and years of impotence, returning to a *normal* sex life may be difficult, for the impotent man *and* for the partner. To add to their difficulties, in many cases the man may require injection therapy, an external management device, or a surgical implant to achieve an erection. With medically prescribed support, he can overcome the effects of his impotence—he will be capable of gaining and maintaining an erection throughout intercourse. However, their renewed attempts at lovemaking may not stand up to their romanticized memories of yesteryear.

Many men remember lovemaking—and the size of their erect penis—much as they would the "fish that got away." They forget that they are no longer twenty-one. Medical intervention can restore an erect penis, but it cannot increase youthful desire and vigor, nor can it make you a better lover than you were before becoming impotent.

Many women are afraid to resume sexual intercourse. One woman told us she was afraid that during their twenty years of abstinence, she'd become a virgin again. Another woman was so tense that her vagina wasn't lubricating and penetration was extremely painful. And many women express their concern about making love to a "fake" or "man-made" penis, not with a man who is *turned on* by her charm and sex appeal. (This is actually not true. The penis is not "fake" or "man-made"; only the blood action has been replaced.)

Couples need time to experiment, to discover a new definition of "normal" that fits their needs and expectations. During this period of adjustment, they will need to be supportive, tender, and understanding; and above all they will need to communicate to one another what they are thinking, feeling, and wanting. We also find that a good sense of humor can help you through many difficult situations. Try to relax, and don't take yourselves too seriously.

Counselors and support groups are very well suited for helping the impotent man and his partner formulate realistic expectations, and for helping them rebuild their relationship.

ADJUSTING TO A NEW WAY OF LOVEMAKING

If you require injection therapy, an external management device, or an implant, you and your partner will need to make some physical and psychological adjustments to your lovemaking. You may need to change your *techniques* as well as the way you relate to one another.

At first, the woman may worry about whether her allure and sex appeal is really arousing her partner. Beth told us that she'd never thought about how her husband's erection had reinforced her feelings about herself until Matt lost that ability.

To help Beth overcome her loss, Matt reassured her that *she* was sexually exciting him. He did this during foreplay with love talk about his feelings and physical pleasures. And as Matt became more aroused, he gradually (and unobtrusively) inflated his implant to simulate a *natural* erection.

New techniques of lovemaking do not come naturally—they come through a lot of trial and error. Eileen was concerned about the "fake" or "man-made" component inside Bruce. Once she even worried that it might be like a dildo. Eileen shared with an I-Anon group her experiences following Bruce's implant surgery:

> "I didn't know how the device would work and Bruce wasn't sure either. The doctor had shown Bruce how to pump it up every day following his surgery to avoid scar tissue from forming. And every day Bruce would say, 'I wonder if I can use this tonight.' Finally I said, 'Shut up. When you find you can use it, let me know.' But there was no one to tell us about this. We simply had to learn from our mistakes. And that's one major reason we started Impotents Anonymous for impotent men and I-Anon for partners—to provide medically sound and realistic information to couples so they wouldn't have to go through what we and thousands of others had to before these support groups were available."
>
> A woman in the front row interrupted, "How can I relax if he wants to make love every night of the week?"
>
> Everyone laughed.
>
> "Well, the novelty does wear off after a while. So you will be able to get back to a normal sex life. Soon we found that we didn't think any more of Bruce's implant than we did of him wearing his glasses, his ring, or his wristwatch. Lovemaking became an automatic thing, his implant became a *natural part of him.*"

In the next room, Bruce was sharing his experiences at an I.A. meeting:

"At first I was a bit clumsy using my implant. We were too concerned with mechanics instead of emotions. I had to be careful not to interrupt our romantic mood by stopping to inflate my device. It wasn't long though until it became second nature. [Some partners often help with the pump as they engage in foreplay.] You know, it's funny, but in some ways my implant is better than Mother Nature. I don't need to worry about premature ejaculation, because my erection lasts as long as I want it. And I've experienced postejaculatory pleasures I never could—even as a young man."

A man seated near the middle of the room raised his hand. "What's the secret to warming up your relationship again?"

"Fortunately," Bruce replied, "Eileen and I were able to maintain good communication between us throughout our entire ordeal. Above all things, our ability to discuss our disappointments, our needs, our worries, and our hopes made the biggest difference in our complete recovery."

BECOMING "COMPLETE" AGAIN

A number of men will have their "natural" potency restored through medical treatment or counseling. Most, however, will need to rely on injection therapy, external management devices, or penile implants to *overcome the effects of their impotence.* For these men, the saying "Once an impotent man, always an impotent man" will always ring true.

Caution—Conservatism—Realism. These are the watchwords for couples recovering from impotence. Be cautious about the decisions you make. Be conservative in your actions. And adopt realistic expectations. Out of your misery can grow opportunity, *if* you take advantage of it.

When a man overcomes the *effects* of his impotence

and is able to satisfy his partner through penile-vaginal intercourse, he has taken a giant step toward restoring his male ego. His sexual success will spill over into all aspects of his life. He will become more self-confident, calmer, less critical, more sharing, and more willing to socialize.

He and his partner can stop living a lie—to their friends and to each other. They no longer have to pretend to be someone other than who they really are. They can laugh and enjoy living again.

THE SECRETS TO YOUR SUCCESS

Remember our five-point formula for your success:

1. *Don't wait,* hoping that things will get better without professional treatment. Impotence is often a symptom of a serious and sometimes life-threatening disease that requires professional treatment.
2. *Do not play doctor* by diagnosing yourself, using logic, and prescribing your own treatment.
3. *Go directly to a urologist* specializing in the diagnosis and treatment of impotence problems.
4. *Act on the specialist's advice.*
5. And remember, *regaining your erection is only the beginning.*

There are new horizons to enjoy. Overcoming the effects of impotence provides you with new opportunities—opportunities to be more expressive in your foreplay, to vocalize your feelings and needs, and to enjoy post-ejaculatory pleasures never before possible.

At last you will have the opportunity to feel like a full man. And your partner will be reassured of your love and respect.

Follow our formula and you, like us and the thousands we've helped, will once again find sexual fulfillment and your happy ending.

11

WHAT SHOULD I DO? LETTERS TO IMPOTENTS ANONYMOUS (I.A.) AND I-ANON

Each week we receive hundreds of letters from people seeking the *truth* about impotence. We should like to share with you their experiences, worries, hopes, and questions, and we'd like to share our answers to them. Many letters address the same types of topics: for example, "Am I really impotent?" "Should I tell my family?" "How can we start to talk about it?" "Does my religion approve of treating impotence?" or "Should I use a particular treatment or device?" Therefore, to help you find the information of most interest to your situation, we've divided the letters into common categories.

In some cases we have corrected the spelling and have deleted extraneous text from the letters. However, we've done our best to preserve the original meaning. The initials, cities, and personal details have been disguised to protect the anonymity of the person writing the inquiry.

AM I REALLY IMPOTENT?

Dear I-Anon:

Thank you for sending me the information about I.A. and I-Anon. My husband and I have been attending our local chapter meetings for nearly nine months and everyone has been very helpful. But now I want to ask you another question.

My husband and I haven't had successful relations for nearly six years. I had to drag him to the first I.A. meeting, but now that he's been attending, I can't get him to do anything about his condition. His urologist says he has poor blood circulation to his penis and he should get an implant. We have piles of literature from manufacturers and stacks of books from the library. We ordered your tape and he's read every article printed on the subject. But he won't do anything about it. Sometimes he gets erections before he wakes up in the morning. He says he isn't sure that he needs the surgery. What should I do?

A. F.
Atlanta, GA

Dear A. F.:

Your husband's obsession with learning everything about impotence is quite common. When the man learns that something can be done, he first becomes enthused. He collects manufacturer's literature, goes to I.A. meetings, and becomes a pretty good authority on the subject. Then fear sets in, and procrastination. Some wait over a year before making a decision. But when the man finally does get his implant, he wonders why he waited so long.

Many organically impotent men get erections during the night. However, they are usually infrequent, of poor quality or short duration. A sleep study conducted by a urologist can provide these answers.

I suggest that you discuss your concerns with your husband and with other partners attending your I-Anon chapter. If necessary, you and your husband may need to visit with his urologist about the situation or see a psychologist for some counseling.

Sounds like you are on the right track. It may just take a little more patience on your part.

Dear Mrs. MacKenzie:

I saw you last week on the "Today" show. I really appreciated how straightforward you answered everyone's questions. It was really nice to get some accurate information for a change.

When I married six years ago, I noticed some problem with impotence. My condition has gotten slightly better since I stopped drinking. But sometimes I can't get stiff enough. I am a recovering alcoholic. I smoke three packs of cigarettes a day.

I don't know if I need help or not. I would respect your opinion.

G. K.
Austin, TX

Dear G. K.:

Apparently your condition has continued over several years. You need to stop fooling yourself and get a professional medical evaluation from a urologist specialist. Only then will you have the correct answers to your questions.

Today there are many alternatives available to help men with chronic physical or psychological impotence. I've enclosed a list of urologists who specialize in the treatment of impotence in your area. You may also want to attend your local I.A. chapter meetings.

Dear Impotents Anonymous:

I received your brochure in the mail. Thank you for answering so quickly. I think my problem may be different from most people you help. Sometimes I have good erections, and other times I lose it before my girl friend is finished. This is very embarrassing to me and I want to know what I can do about it. Do you really think I'm impotent? Do you think vitamins will help?

M. V.
Seattle, WA

Dear M. V.:

From your letter, it appears that you do have an erectile problem. Recommending a course of treatment, such as vitamins, would be premature.

First you need to see a urologist specialist who can correctly diagnose the cause of your problem. Nearly 75 percent of impotence can be attributed to physical problems. Impotence may be a symptom of a serious disease process, even a life-threatening one. You should not continue to put off seeing a urologist specialist. Enclosed is a list of urologists in your area.

IS IT IN MY HEAD?

Dear Eileen MacKenzie:

I was married to my husband five years ago. Even in the beginning he wasn't very interested in having sex. But during the last two years, he has avoided me more and more. He works all day and goes to school at night. Most of the time he says he's too tired. He is under a lot of pressure lately. I think he needs to go to a sex therapist. But he won't even talk with me about it. What should I do?

P. W.
Chicago, IL

Dear P. W.:

It is imperative that you and your husband stop playing doctor—stop making excuses for his impotence. Bruce and I had every reason to feel the same way you do. We sought counseling for several years. But we were wrong. Only when we went to a urologist specialist did we find that Bruce had a physical problem. You cannot determine that without a medical evaluation.

Since only 25 to 35 percent of impotence can be explained with psychological causes, I encourage you to consult with a urologist specialist for a complete medical evaluation.

Dear I.A.:

I am thirty-seven years old and have been impotent all of my life. I recently married a woman who was aware of my condition prior to our getting married. But now she wants a resolution of my problem as soon as possible. I went to a urologist who told me my condition was not physical. He would not give me an implant. I have been in psychotherapy for over two years and my therapist thinks an implant is the best option for me.

Would you please tell me who would be willing to perform the surgery even though I do not have a physical problem? This is causing marital difficulties, which we believe would not be present if the problem were solved.

E. Y.
Grand Island, NE

Dear E. Y.:

Some doctors will not implant men with psychogenic impotence—not under any circumstances. Others will do so on a psychologist's recommendations. We have made several inquiries to urologist specialists in your area. We did not give your name to them. Enclosed is a list of urologists who will consider doing your surgery.

Dear I-Anon:

I want to thank you very much for the information that you sent to me on Impotents Anonymous.

The various bits of information gave me direction, and my only trouble was all psychological! I tried too hard! Thank you again, and now I can make it on my own.

H. R. S.
Ohio

Dear Bruce and Eileen:

About two years ago, I noticed that my sexual drive and ability to perform were deteriorating. I figured that it was a problem that would pass in time. It didn't. So a year ago I went to see a doctor and told him about my problem. He said I was physically okay and made me an appointment with a psychiatrist. He blamed my impotence on my wife and asked that she come with me for our counseling sessions. I'm thoroughly convinced that my head is on straight and that there is something physically wrong with me that the original doctor I consulted did not detect.

I am in the Air Force. I think that I'm in pretty good health. I don't smoke at all, I don't drink a lot, and I don't feel overly stressed in my work. I also exercise regularly every other day. The only other problems I have besides frequent impotence is a frequent fatigued feeling and sometimes an extremely upset stomach—especially after I drink wine in the evening.

Can you arm me with some knowledge about my problem? I'd really like to check in with the doctor again, but I'd like to have some idea of what he should be checking for.

U. O.
Orlando, FL

Dear U. O.:

Unless you went to a urologist who specializes in impotence and took the tests required to eliminate physical impotence as a cause, you cannot be certain that you have a psychological problem.

Most urologist specialists will do a complete physical examination including blood tests for diabetes, hormone levels, liver function, and so forth. In addition, they may recommend tests to determine if you have good-quality erections during the night—most men will have three to five of these every night. If you do have good-quality erections at night, you probably do have a psychological problem. If, however, you do not, your doctor will want to run additional tests to determine the physical cause.

Whatever the cause, today there are many options available: medical treatment, penile injections, external management devices, and penile implants.

We recommend that you see a urologist specialist as soon as possible.

AM I TOO OLD?

Dear Impotents Anonymous:

I am sixty years old and I was told by my urologist that impotence is something that happens with age. I began to wonder about his advice when I read about you in *The Wall Street Journal* article. So I went to a urologist specialist and he found that I had a vascular problem. Now I'm taking a vasodilator and I have quit smoking. This solved my problem.

My wife couldn't believe there was an organization

like yours that gave such good information. We're leaving for our second honeymoon.

B. L.
Danville, IN

Dear Impotents Anonymous:

On Thursday April 30, 1987, I saw three men interviewed on the "Today" show about their impotence problems, and your address was given at the end of that interview.

I am fifty-nine years old, married for twenty-five years, and I am experiencing some of the same problems that these men spoke about. I do not have a stressful occupation, but I did work at a nuclear power plant for ten years.

There is a record of diabetes in my family. My father and one brother have the disease but as yet I have not been diagnosed as having diabetes.

Consultations with my family doctor have given me no answers except that he thought all men have some degree of impotence problems as they get older.

Please advise me on what further steps I should take to resolve my problems.

D. K.
Pittsburgh, PA

Dear D. K.:

Age in and of itself does not cause impotence. Many eighty-year-old men enjoy an active sex life, while some twenty-year-olds have severe erectile problems. It's true that the aging process, which includes problems such as hardening of the arteries, can contribute to an impotence problem.

Before drawing any conclusions, however, you should consult with a urologist specialist who has the expertise and equipment required to make an accurate medical diagnosis.

Dear Impotents Anonymous:

I am a man seventy-six years old who has enjoyed sex all my life. About four years ago I lost my erectile ability. So I went to a urologist. After an examination, he found a blocked artery on the right side of my penis. He recommended I get a penile implant.

But right after that, I had a five-artery heart bypass. I have talked to my heart doctor about having this operation and he said he could not see anything wrong with having it done.

At my age, now seventy-six, do you think it foolish to have the operation, or is there some other method or way this problem could be handled?

I have lady friends around my age who would enjoy sex with me. So I feel embarrassed when I am around them. Any advice or help on this matter would be very appreciated.

A. J.
Dallas, TX

Dear A. J.:

Thank you for your letter. You are by no means foolish to consider overcoming your impotence. The oldest man known by us to have had the implant surgery is eighty-nine. However, before deciding on the surgery, you should know that there are other treatments available to you—for example, the PEP self-injection program and external management devices.

I would suggest you consult further with your urologist regarding treatment. If your cardiologist sees no problem with the surgery, an implant may be the way to go.

DOES MY RELIGION APPROVE OF TREATING IMPOTENCE?

Dear I-Anon:

My husband and I were married five years ago and we have not been able to consummate our marriage. He went to a urologist and he found 100 percent organic damage to his vascular system. Injection therapy and external management devices are not appropriate. The doctor recommended an implant.

The Roman Catholic religion cannot bless our marriage if it is not consummated. But will our faith allow this surgical procedure?

I. V.
Newark, NJ

Dear I. V.:

To answer your letter, I'd like to quote Dr. David Kelly, professor of theology at Duquesne University, Worcester, MA. Father Kelly says, "I have found no work done by the Roman Catholic Church or a Catholic moral theologian who criticizes or forbids penile implants. It seems to be correcting, in a perfectly valid way, a defect in the man's genital system. . . . It seems to me that contemporary Roman Catholic theology recognizes sexuality as a gift of a loving God. This is a way in which medicine can restore that gift to human beings who, for one reason or another, have lost normal sexual functioning."

Dear Impotents Anonymous:

I am scheduled for a penile implant next month. But now I have some qualms from a religious point of view. Would God approve of such surgery? Would God approve of my resuming sexual intercourse again? I am a single man.

Y. C.
White Plains, NY

Dear Y. C.:

From your letter I cannot tell what religion you practice. So I will tell you what we know.

Dr. Walter Jacob, Senior Rabbi of Rodef-Shalom Congregation and Shamen of the Responsa Committee dealing with Jewish law of the Central Conference of American Rabbis, says, "Penile implants would simply be taken as a surgical procedure that would help someone. It does not remove anything. . . . There is no one—orthodox, conservative, or reform—who would have any hesitancy about that."

The Reverend Paul Schrading, council director of the Western Pennsylvania Conference of United Methodists, is unaware of any position on penile implants by either his own church or any other Protestant denomination. "My personal opinion would be that any scientific advances that would enable someone to fulfill a love relationship in marriage and make it more satisfying would be generally favorable."

Dr. David Kelly, associate professor of theology at Duquesne University, says he has found no work done by the Roman Catholic Church or a Catholic moral theologian who criticizes or forbids penile implants.

We've also been told by a Baptist minister of some thirty years that the Baptists don't reject this type of surgery.

In addition, our mailman, who is also a preacher for a small Protestant sect, asked for our literature to keep at their church and ministerial school.

We have not heard of any Western religion that objects to penile implant surgery.

HOW CAN WE START TO TALK ABOUT OUR PROBLEM?

Dear Eileen MacKenzie:

I saw you last week on the "Sally Jessy Raphael" show.

My husband is in his twenties. He is very caring, but he couldn't care less about having sex. And when I bring it up, he doesn't want to talk about it. Would you please tell me what I can do?

S. F.
Boca Raton, FL

Dear S. F.:

I suggest that you attend an I-Anon meeting to help you cope with this problem. You will learn a great deal from partners who have experienced problems similar to yours. After attending a meeting, tell your husband that you sought help so you could be a better partner to him.

It's important for you to understand that he probably feels a lot of fear, anger, and guilt about this problem. His ego is wounded. Seeking help on your own may help him face his problem, and it won't add additional guilt.

You and he both need to know that today, no man need remain chronically impotent. There is hope.

LETTER 1

Dear Impotents Anonymous:

Do we have troubles? Neither of us can address the troubles. Would you please send me some information about impotence.

O. M.
Tucson, AZ

Dear O. M.:

I suggest you get our videotape in which Bruce and I discuss the experiences we went through. Perhaps this will serve as an icebreaker. If you have not consulted with a urologist specialist, you should do so immediately to find out what is causing your impotence. Impotence can be a symptom of a serious medical problem, which, if left untreated, could even be life-threatening.

In addition, you may wish to consult with a psychologist or marriage counselor to help you with your communication problems. Impotence can place a severe strain on a relationship, and often counseling helps.

LETTER 2

Dear Eileen MacKenzie:

Thank you so much for the information you sent. We got your tape, watched it, and then talked about it. As a result of your referral, I went to a urologist specialist who found that I have diabetes, severe blood-pressure problems, and complications from the medicine I'm taking. I've decided to get an implant.

My wife and I are seeing a marriage counselor and our tension has gone down considerably.

Thanks for caring.

O. M.
Tucson, AZ

Dear I-Anon:

We got married three years ago. From the beginning, my husband had difficulty with intercourse. And now he's ceased altogether. My husband is an alcoholic, but he is not drinking. He blames everyone, especially me, for his problems. I'm very down and depressed. He has a bad temper and sometimes becomes very violent. But he's nice most of the time. Please tell me what I can do.

M. N.
York, PA

Dear M. N.:

Most chronically impotent men feel embarrassment, fear, anger, and frustration with the loss of their sexual abilities. It sounds as though your husband is reacting more strongly to his problem than most do. Some of his fear and anger may subside if he knew that one in ten men in the United States is chronically impotent. He is not alone. In addition, he might be encouraged to know that nearly every impotent man can be helped. He should see a urologist specialist right away to determine the cause of his impotence.

I strongly suggest you find an AL-Anon group to help you cope with your nondrinking alcoholic. You might consider getting some counseling as well. There is more than impotence going on in your relationship.

SHOULD I TELL MY FAMILY ABOUT MY IMPOTENCE?

Dear I-Anon:

My husband is going to get an implant next month. But we don't know what to tell our children. We're afraid that they might think he has cancer or something if we hide the reason for his surgery. Neither of us want them to worry. What should we do?

B. A.
Oklahoma City, OK

Dear B. A.:

Bruce and I had several discussions about this before telling our children. We finally decided that honesty was the best policy—we were tired of living a lie with our closest loved ones. At the time, our youngest was eighteen and all five were married.

We called all of our children and their spouses together and told them why Bruce was going to the hospital—to get his implant.

We found that disclosing our secret drew us closer together. The boys began to realize that this could happen to them. And the girls were interested in Eileen's concerns about the importance of intimate lovemaking. Our children were very understanding and supportive.

Two days after Bruce's surgery, everyone gathered at our home and called him long distance.

We believe you should be totally honest with older children.

(The problem might be theirs in later life.)

Dear Impotents Anonymous:

I thought I would share an interesting series of events with you.

Several months ago I read about I.A. in our local paper. I wrote to you to get some information for my father, who is a minister. I thought he might be able to use it with his parishioners.

A few weeks after I sent the information to him, my mother called to ask how I knew that my father and she had the problem. It took me ten minutes to convince her that I didn't know.

Now that I do though, we've grown even closer. Next month I'm flying out to visit them. This has opened doors of communication on a deeper loving level.

Father is using the injection treatments, very successfully.

I just thought you might enjoy hearing about this surprising coincidence.

C. Y.
Lexington, KY

Dear Impotents Anonymous:

As I write this letter, I am in tears. Over the last year my father has become more and more depressed. He's very bad tempered and difficult to deal with. Every time I try to talk with him, he shuts me out.

Last week I visited with him and he had a few drinks too many. It was then that he told me about his problem with impotence. He is ashamed, depressed, and in despair.

He is a widower and he had to end a relationship with a lady because he couldn't pursue a marriage.

What can I do?

S. C.
Billings, MT

Dear S. C.:

Your father is very lucky that he has a daughter who cares so much about him.

I encourage you to get your father to a urologist specialist as soon as possible. He needs a complete medical evaluation to determine what is causing his impotence problem.

With proper diagnosis and treatment, it's almost certain that he can overcome the effects of his impotence and once again have a satisfactory relationship with a woman.

Dear Impotents Anonymous:

I'm in my late sixties and my son is in his forties. We both are diabetic and we are both impotent. We have very good marriages and at one time had a very good sex life.

Amazingly, at approximately the same time, our wives—who are very close—noticed a difference in our attitudes. They discussed the similarities with one another and finally confronted each of us individually.

Between the four of us, with the helpful input from your organization we've worked out solutions to our problems, and the whole thing drew our family closer together.

P. D.
New York, NY

WHAT IS THE BEST WAY FOR ME TO OVERCOME THE EFFECTS OF MY IMPOTENCE?

Dear Impotents Anonymous:

Do you have any personal knowledge about the ——— device? Is it credible? Does it have a record of acceptance? Is the manufacturer reliable? If I have erections during sleep, can I have a physical problem?

K. L.
Baton Rouge, LA

Dear K. L.:

Our National Medical Advisor, Dr. Myron Murdock, informs us that a person with erectile dysfunction can have erections during sleep. Every night, a man with normal erectile function will have three to five erections of good intensity lasting fifteen to thirty minutes each. If there is a decrease in frequency, intensity, or duration—a quantitative loss—then the man could have a physical problem. A medically controlled sleep study can best determine if you are having normal erections.

With regard to the device you asked about, we've enclosed the manufacturer's literature for your review. They are a very reputable company. I do advise, however, that you consult with a urologist specialist about your condition. It's premature to be thinking about a device before you know the origin of your problem.

Dear Impotents Anonymous:

Please send me information on malleable penile implants. I live hundreds of miles from the U.S. and I will have to travel a long distance to have surgery.

K. F.

Dear K. F.:

Enclosed is the information you requested on malleable penile implants. Since you do not have a urologist specialist in your area, we suggest you call us collect and talk to Bruce about your situation. We are concerned that you get sound advice before you decide on surgery.

Dear Bruce MacKenzie:

I am the pastor of a church. I can get good erections; however, I cannot maintain them long enough. From the information you sent me earlier this year, I believe I should try an external management device. Do you recommend the one made by ———?

S. L.
Collingswood, NJ

Dear S. L.:

From what you describe, the ——— external management device may be just what you need. I must caution you, however, not to play doctor and diagnose your problem. Impotence can be the symptom of a serious medical problem. Please contact a urologist specialist before you decide what is the best way to overcome your impotence problem.

Dear I-Anon:

My husband had open heart surgery following a heart attack. He's taking medication for rapid heartbeat and high blood pressure. Because of his heart condition, I'm concerned about his having penile implant surgery.

But he feels so belittled; it's not good for him. I don't think he would go to a sex therapist or to counseling. He would read some of your literature, however. So please send me some information on his condition.

K. F.
St. Louis, MO

Dear K. F.:

I'm sure that your urologist specialist will work closely with your husband's cardiologist with regard to recommending surgery. If the cardiologist feels the implant surgery is appropriate, then I would not be overly concerned. Many men with your husband's problem have been helped in this way.

You should know, however, if surgery would be ruled out there are alternatives to a penile implant—injection therapy and external management devices, for example. You may wish to discuss your concerns and these options with your urologist specialist.

Dear Bruce MacKenzie:

I was a survivor of the Holocaust. I am a diabetic and two years ago, I had open heart surgery. Also, I am impotent. But I took a chance and had a penile implant. I'm here to tell you, everything is worth it. Anyone who doesn't seek help is a loser. Life is too short. You should enjoy life any way you can.

S. S.

Dear S. S.

Your letter gave Bruce and me great pleasure. We are to be in your area to open a chapter of I.A. in three weeks at ——— Hospital. Dr. ——— is the urologist medical advisor. If you would be interested in attending and be willing to share your experiences, I know everyone would enjoy hearing you. If you do come to the meeting please introduce yourself to Bruce and me.

Dear S. S.

It was a pleasure to meet you and hear your story at the meeting. Dr. ———, Bruce, and I are very grateful for your offer to be the lay coordinator for this chapter. It is people like yourself who can do so much to help other impotent men overcome their fears and make decisions. Enclosed is material to guide you at future meetings.

Again, our sincere thanks to you.

Dear Impotents Anonymous:

Two years ago I had a colostomy to remove a malignant tumor. The doctor prescribed radiology treatments, but halfway through the treatments I began having erection problems. At the end of the treatments, I could not have an erection, even at night.

The doctor also says I have retrograde ejaculation. But I'm not sure I understand this. He wants me to get an implant. I am seventy-four years old, very healthy, and play tennis twice a week. Do you think I should get the implant?

I. T.
Huntington, WV

Dear I. T.:

It sounds like you've made a remarkable recovery from your surgery and radiation therapy.

Retrograde ejaculation means that when you ejaculate your semen, some or all of the fluid squirts into your bladder instead of out of your penis. This is not harmful. You will expel the semen the next time you urinate.

The colostomy and/or the radiation therapy probably damaged the nerves that serve your penis and the blood vessels going to your penis. The penile implant is an excellent method for overcoming your impotence. However, you may wish to discuss penile injection therapy and external management devices with your urologist specialist.

Dear Impotents Anonymous:

I am forty-one years old and have had erection problems for the past two years. I heard on TV that there is an injection which will cause an erection. Is the solution injected into the urethra? I would ask a urologist, only I'm afraid he'd try to sell me on an implant. Could you send me some information about this?

D. F.
Houston, TX

Dear D. F.:

The papaverine/Regitine penile erection program (PEP) works well for many men with physical or psychogenic impotence. Using a small needle, the medication is injected into the base of the penis. Within five to fifteen minutes you will have an erection that lasts an hour or more. Your urologist specialist can give you the injection in his office to see if the medication will work for you.

A new, more expensive drug called prostaglandin E_1 is available for men who cannot tolerate papaverine/Regitine injections, which sometimes disturb liver function.

You cannot obtain these drugs yourself. You must see a urologist specialist who will determine if the drug will help your condition and who will determine the correct dosage.

Please remember that, subject to your medical situation, the choice of treatment is yours. You should consult with a urologist specialist who is willing to work with your needs.

Dear Eileen MacKenzie:

My husband has hardening of the arteries. He consulted with a urologist who offered him the PEP program but he did not favor this. He doesn't want an implant either. What he wants is a *miracle!* Also, I know he is concerned about money. We have insurance, but it won't pay for everything.

J. C.
Albuquerque, NM

Dear J. C.:

As your husband is reluctant to use penile injections or to get an implant, he might consider using an external management device. Many men, and couples, are very happy with them. These devices are relatively inexpensive, and some come with a thirty-day money-back guarantee. It might be worth a try if your urologist recommends it.

Dear Impotents Anonymous:

My husband has had an impotence problem for four and a half years. He is a dentist. A year and a half ago, he began using the PEP program, and now we have a three-month-old baby boy. We just wanted your newsletter readers to know that penile injections do not adversely affect your fertility. We are a very happy family.

K. S.
Los Angeles, CA

Dear K. S.:

We are all delighted at Headquarters to know of your happiness and congratulate you on the birth of your son. Being a mother and grandmother, I know the joy a child can bring to a family.

Your news will definitely be included in our newsletter, and we thank you for being willing to share it. I know it will be encouraging and helpful for many readers.

Dear Impotents Anonymous:

Diabetes has gradually decreased my ability to get an erection. Do you have a method that will help without getting an implant?

I read an article in a medical magazine that there is an injection (shot) that will help.

Please advise.

T. B.
Tulsa, OK

Dear T. B.:

Today there are many alternative treatments for overcoming the effects of impotence: penile injections, external management devices, and penile implants.

Before you decide what method is best for you, I encourage you to attend an I.A. meeting in your community. There you can discuss—with men who have "walked in your shoes"—your concerns and questions. And you can discuss many alternatives with the I.A. chapter Urologist Medical Advisor.

Dear Impotents Anonymous:

I'm impotent to a certain extent. I wish to try the vacuum constrictor devices that the FDA has approved. Two versions are relatively new; they involve placing a plastic cylinder over the shaft of the penis, pumping out the air to create a vacuum, producing an erection. I am interested in buying the device. Please send me the information and the price of the device. Thank you.

S. C.
Winneconne, WI

Dear S. C.:

I am enclosing a pamphlet regarding a vacuum constrictor device. Also, other material about external management devices is enclosed. They work well for many people.

However, before making any decision regarding the use of such a device, you should consult with a urologist who specializes in impotence. You need to know the cause of your erection problem. Remember that there are more treatments available today than in the past. You need the one most appropriate for your special case.

Dear Impotents Anonymous:

Thank God you're there!! It's difficult to get enough information about impotence.

I read an article in *50 Plus* (September 1986) saying you have information. I work for a hospital that has a urology department, but I'd like to know a lot more about penile prostheses.

Also tell me if there is an Impotents Anonymous chapter near me.

N. F.
Joplin, MO

Dear N. F.:

There are several types of penile prostheses, including the semirigid, malleable, hinged, self-contained, and fully inflatable. All of these implants work well, and partners report that they cannot tell the difference from a nonimplanted penis.

I suggest that you attend the local Impotents Anonymous meeting to find out more about these devices from the Urologist Medical Advisor and from men who already have received an implant. Enclosed are several brochures for your review.

Dear I.A.:

I am interested in organizing an Impotents Anonymous chapter in my area.

I had a penile implant three years ago. I am a very active sixty-nine-year-old male. My doctor warned me I may need to use a special bicycle seat because cycling is my special interest.

I not only proved a standard racing-type seat could be used; I have bicycle toured more than 10,000 miles since my operation.

I want to help other men who are hurting. I know there are men my age and younger men who need help. I believe there are more closeted impotent males in America than there were closeted homosexuals. We must bring them to the surface so they can get help. There is help for every man who needs help. I believe the penile implant is the answer when all else fails.

G. C.

(Location omitted to maintain anonymity)

Dear G. C.

Your delightful letter was read with great interest by Bruce and me, and your enthusiasm is welcomed by us.

I enclose a pamphlet that gives information on starting chapters of Impotents Anonymous and I-Anon, together with other materials describing our organization and its purposes and goals. You will note that it is a mandatory requirement that each chapter has a Urologist Medical Advisor who is a professional member of the Impotence Institute of America together with one or more lay coordinators (a man/men and woman/women who have experienced the trauma of impotence in their lives). It is these lay coordinators who can relate to the attendees at a meeting and who are of such help and encouragement. They have "walked in the shoes"!

Your letter came at a most opportune moment. There is a chapter starting up in your area, and we shall appreciate your contacting Dr. ———, and offering your help. I know he will be delighted to have your assistance. If you know of others like yourself who would be interested in helping, please ask them to write to us at Headquarters, 119 South Ruth Street, Department Y, Maryville, TN 37801.

I must inform you that, although for your particular case you have found the penile implant to be the answer, we believe that people should be informed of all means of treatment. For some the answer may be the injection program, therapy, or an external management device. Our purpose is to educate people as to causes and all treatments available, and to offer both emotional and informational support *without bias* to men and their partners in coping with impotence.

Dear Impotents Anonymous:

We just celebrated our fourteenth wedding anniversary and I just wanted to write you a special "thank you" letter. The operation performed by the doctor you recommended has turned out to be excellent. I have only the utmost gratitude.

After doing without sex for many years, it was great to know we could at last express our feelings for one another. We both had forgotten just how wonderful sex used to be to us.

My husband was concerned with the length, but now he has changed his mind; the length couldn't be any better. The performance is great. In fact, now when he reaches his climax, we don't even have to stop after the climax as in the past, because his penis does not go soft. We don't have to stop until I want to, and that's a *great feeling.* We are also able to achieve other positions with no problem and no difficulties in climaxing.

We have been through a lot together. When I took my marriage vows, I promised to love and cherish him through sickness and in health, for better or worse. And believe me, I have been through some tough times with him. So from two happy people, we say, God bless you and many thanks!

H. N.
Washington, DC

WHAT CAN IMPOTENTS ANONYMOUS AND I-ANON DO FOR ME?

Dear Impotents Anonymous:

Thank you for your fine work and invaluable information. Before I started attending my local I.A. chapter, I had an attitude of resigned acceptance. My condition fostered all sorts of negative emotions: anger, frustration, resentment, and discouragement.

Now I'm being treated for very long-term impotence. Thanks to your efforts, a new feeling is emerging: hope.

D. M.
Elizabeth, NJ

Dear Impotents Anonymous:

I wanted to let your newsletter readers know the problems I've had getting treatment for my impotence. One doctor took my money and left the country. Another doctor tells me I should get an implant, but he cannot give me the name of one of his patients to talk to. His nurse calls me periodically trying to get me to schedule my surgery.

Attending I.A. meetings, I learned from the urologist and others that there are many more types of implants than either of the previous doctors had told me about. I wonder how many other sufferers have given up because of receiving similar treatment? All of this was unnecessary and expensive. I've lost faith in the medical profession.

T. P.
New York, NY

Dear T. P.:

Similar experiences to yours take place all too frequently around the country. And many men do become discouraged and return to the closet to suffer in silence.

You know you have the wrong doctor if he does not let you talk to men who have gone through the surgery, if he does not talk about all treatments available, and if he tries to rush you into a decision about surgery. You need to be very sure and content with the surgical option before making that decision.

I'm glad the I.A. chapter and Urologist Medical Advisor have been helpful to you. Perhaps now you can begin to resolve your situation.

Dear Impotents Anonymous:

I got the information about your program from Dr. Art Ulene's TV program. How much are the meetings? Are meetings male and female mixed? What are the requirements for membership?

After seeing two urologists, I have two different paths to follow. Do you suggest I see a psychologist? I'm interested in getting any help. I've been impotent for three years.

E. L.
Little Rock, AR

Dear E. L.:

There is no charge for an Impotents Anonymous or I-Anon meeting. They are absolutely free. You may make a voluntary contribution to support your local chapter, if you so desire.

The majority of meetings are open for both men and partners. Any member, however, may ask for a closed meeting of men or partners. The only requirement for membership is that you attended a meeting. A desire to learn about and discuss the problem of impotence will help you. We keep no membership list because your anonymous membership is kept absolutely confidential.

If you would like a referral to a psychologist, we can provide you with the name of one practicing in your area.

Dear I-Anon:

Thank God I found you. Before I received your tape, my husband refused to discuss his problem with me. I'd been groping in the dark for five years, talking to urologists and therapists untrained in impotence. Through an article in a local paper, I located I.A.

My husband had denied he had a problem. He is gone many months out of the year because of his work. He'd constantly shelved the problem, promising to "work on it." The frustration had become almost unbearable.

Because of your information, my husband has agreed to see a urologist on your list. He's agreed to look at the tape and read the information when he returns home.

Now we have someone to turn to. God has used you in a beautiful way.

T. N.
Grand Rapids, MI

Dear Impotents Anonymous:

I had colon surgery and lengthy radiation treatments. I read the article about you in *The Wall Street Journal.* Please send me information. Can a similar information center be set up in my city? I would make myself available to help with such an endeavor.

M. P.
Rochester, MN

Dear M. P.:

Each of our Impotents Anonymous and I-Anon chapters has a Urologist Medical Advisor and a lay coordinator. Many chapters also have a Mental Health Professional advisor. Enclosed is some additional information about Impotents Anonymous and the names of our professional members in your city. You may wish to talk to them about setting up an I.A. chapter.

Dear Impotents Anonymous:

I believe that my attendance at some I.A. chapter meetings last year was directly responsible for my impotence being completely cured. I am now able to function as many as three times in one night!

My main cause of impotence was lack of penile blood pressure due to a narrowing of that very small artery that supplies the blood for an erection.

After a complete evaluation by a urologist you recommended, I decided to get a penile implant. The total cost was a little over $10,000 but my insurance covered 80 percent of the costs.

S. F.
Jackson, TN

Dear Eileen and Bruce:

In reading your newsletter stating that interest has been shown in opening 236 chapters—you really must be busy.

I enjoyed my four-hour session with Dr. Murdock, your National Medical Advisor. He was most informative.

Our I.A. meetings are finally getting to the point where the lay audience is assuming many of the responsibilities. The lay coordinators are doing a really good job in their take-over. We are pleased that our chapter has initiated the Friendly Visitor service. They decided to have members of the chapter visit men in the hospital following surgery for implants.

M. B., M.D.
(Location omitted to maintain anonymity)

Dear M. B.:

It was with great interest that Bruce and I read your letter about the start of your Friendly Visitor service. This information is to be included in the next issue of our newsletter, and we hope other groups will start a similar program. Bruce knows only too well the need for support during a hospital stay. Congratulations. You and your group are doing a wonderful job.

Mr. and Mrs. Bruce MacKenzie:

Thank you for your response to my previous letter in your mailbag. I read your article in our publication, *Urol-*

ogy, saying that nicotine and smoking can contribute to impotence. I think the information is most interesting. I learned something. I will introduce this into my practice.

L. K., M.D.
Richmond, VA

Dear Abby:

An article you had in the *Rocky Mountain News* in Denver, CO, a year ago about Impotents Anonymous may have saved my life as I had just about given up on anything. But this gave me hope.

At that time, I had spent several thousand dollars and two years of my life trying to find a solution to my impotence.

I urge you to reprint the name and address of I.A./I-Anon: 119 South Ruth Street, Maryville, TN 37801.

I thank you with all my heart. Impotence is a joke until it happens to you.

M. B.
Evergreen, CO

Dear Impotents Anonymous and I-Anon:

You opened up a whole new world to me and others who read the material on impotence you were nice enough to send along.

After several weeks of soul-searching, I called apprehensively. I was captivated by Bruce's helpful attitude and superior knowledge on the subject of impotence. Recent medical developments have leaped ahead in alleviating impotence.

I decided to go to Impotents Anonymous headquarters to personally investigate the situation. Bruce and Eileen could not have been more helpful or cooperative. They really "knocked themselves out" for me.

My wife and I attended an I.A. meeting that literally was a "revelation." Attending were implant recipients (both inflatable and semirigid) extolling the wonders of their rediscovered sexual activities. The wives of the recipients were "bragging about the new joys of their new 'bedroom benders'—where previously only conversation reigned." Also, a well-known urologist experienced in implant procedures answered all medical questions.

After meeting with and undergoing testing by the same urologist, my implant decision was made.

It's been several months since the procedure, and I have entered into the "Bold New World." *Bruce and Eileen were marvelous in their total giving of themselves.*

I.A. and I-Anon are most fortunate in having such a caring and knowledgeable couple as Bruce and Eileen steering this worthy organization in the proper direction.

V. B.
Chula Vista, CA

Dear Eileen:

I have had this terrible situation and kept it a dark secret for fifteen years or so. It was not until I heard of I.A. and went to a couple of meetings that I realized that I am not alone in the world.

Also, through I.A. I learned that it is possible for an ordinary person—one of modest means—to get help. So I am happy to announce to you that I am scheduled for surgery late in July.

If this all works out, as I hope and expect that it will, I will be grateful to you and I.A. for the rest of my life. Believe me, the last few years haven't been pleasant.

F. S.
Fort Wayne, IN

Dear Eileen MacKenzie:

I thank you for the much needed information. You have given hope to me and my wife. Thanks one more time. Also I am asking you to please mail me names and phone numbers of urologists, psychologists, and psychiatrists in my area, if possible. God bless you.

S. B.
Laconia, NH

Dear Impotents Anonymous:

I caught a brief portion of your interview segment on NBC's "Today" last week.

Please send me information or details where I can learn more about impotence. I thought there was no answer to my problem. No one else ever mentioned they had such a condition. Thank you for your consideration.

B. L.
Cleveland, OH

Dear Impotents Anonymous:

I am writing in regard to the excellent program feature on NBC's "Today" show earlier last week. While I did not have the opportunity to view it personally, my wife of twenty-seven years did, and she thought the information and the men who spoke were superb. She felt it should be shown again as a Public Service Announcement.

I am interested in whatever information that may be available for myself, as well as for many of my customers. I am a fifty-three-year-old registered pharmacist and I encounter many of the problems mentioned in the course of a day's work. Most men do not know where to get the proper help.

Also, is there a support group for women? Many

questions come from women who are worried about their husbands, their marriages, etc. I'd like to be able to tell them all about your program and how to get help.

I never realized just how much unhappiness was being caused for so many. My wife said the TV program stated there were millions of men afflicted.

C. H., P.D.
Allentown, PA

Dear C. H.:

We are pleased to know your wife thought well of the impotence segment on the "Today" show. In the United States there are at least 10 million men affected by this problem, and there are many millions more worldwide.

I enclose a number of pamphlets that give basic information concerning impotence. You may wish to give these to those people who ask you for help. If you would like to have more, please let us know.

There is a support program, I-Anon, for partners of impotent men. Meetings are held usually at the same time as Impotents Anonymous meetings. Some meetings are joint, and others separate, depending on the attendees' wishes. Enclosed is a list of meetings held in your area to which people may go in complete anonymity.

People who wish information from our Headquarters may write to us at 119 South Ruth Street, Department Y, Maryville, TN 37801.

If we can be of further assistance, please do not hesitate to contact us.

Dear Bruce MacKenzie:

As long as I have been a doctor, the problem of impotence has been of great interest to me. Evaluation of patients and differential diagnosis of the complaint require sympathy and tact, perhaps best stated by pointing out that one must be human first, physician next, and urologist last.

I am grateful for the opportunity of membership in this organization, which is filling a real need. And I will do my best for any patients who seek my help.

A. M., M.D.
Boston, MA

Dear Impotents Anonymous:

I just watched the "Today" show about impotence.

For years, I have been unable to have a proper erection, and now none. A year ago I went through a divorce after twenty-six years of marriage. My wife thought I had a girlfriend, our [her] love died, and she wanted out. I still love her and hurt very much because I lost her.

I'm still single and probably will remain so because of my problem.

If there is help for me, I sure need it and want it.

The "Today" show didn't say what you have to offer in the way of help.

J. M.
Norfolk, NE

Dear J. M.:

Impotents Anonymous for impotent men and I-Anon for the partners are nonprofit organizations dedicated to providing medically accurate information about chronic impotence to anyone requesting that information.

I want to say to you that there is help available for you. There is no reason for you to remain chronically impotent. I have enclosed a list of urologist specialists in your area and I encourage you to contact one immediately.

I'VE LOST ALL SEXUAL DESIRE, WHAT SHOULD I DO?

Dear I-Anon:

I heard about your organization on a TV show. But I am the one who is impotent, not my husband. I have been hospitalized three times for depression. I've had shock treatment and now I'm on medication. My husband loves me, but I have no desire for sex. He's very good to me. Please tell me what treatments are available for women with impotence.

B. W.
Greensboro, NC

Dear B. W.:

First of all, you should not play doctor by assuming that you are impotent, or that your depression is causing your impotence. You may have another physical problem. You should get a complete medical evaluation from a gynecologist.

One of our medical advisors told us that when a woman lacks sexual desire, it usually is a psychological problem. This symptom is frequently associated with chronic depression. Perhaps one of a number of antidepressant medications available today might improve this situation, but don't do anything without professional direction.

You should consult with your psychiatrist about this problem.

Dear I-Anon:

I've been married three years and it's been difficult from the day we got married. I love my husband and I want to stay with him. However, his lack of interest is getting to me.

He's still in school and we don't have a lot of money. He is not impotent, but I saw you on a television talk show and I thought you could help.

W. S.
Boulder, CO

Dear W. S.:

From what you describe, I don't believe your husband has an impotence problem (the inability to gain and maintain an erection). However, you do need help to improve your relationship. You both should seek counseling. If he refuses to seek help, you should consult with a marriage counselor or sex therapist.

Many colleges provide university clinics for students—at a very reasonable rate. This may be a starting point. You may also wish to check with your county medical society or county health department to see if there is a counseling service that is free or priced according to your ability to pay. Most communities support such programs.

Dear I-Anon:

My husband is involved with alcohol but he is going to AA. I left him once for several months after he beat me. But I went back when he promised to stop his drinking. Now I think that I am impotent because I've lost all desire. Do you think I should get counseling?

L. C.
Shreveport, LA

Dear L. C.:

First you should see a gynecologist to see if you do have a physical problem causing you to lose sexual desire. From the situation you describe, though, I'm not surprised that you feel the way you do. Many wives of alcoholics, especially battered wives, do not feel sexually attracted to their partners.

I suggest that you seek counseling from a battered wife organization such as Victims Anonymous or Batterers Anonymous. In addition, you may wish to attend an AL-Anon meeting.

Dear I-Anon:

Does your organization deal with women who have lost their desire for sex or who can no longer have orgasms? If you do, please send me some information.

K. H.
Lansing, MI

Dear K. H.:

I regret that we only deal with male impotence. Our National Medical Advisor suggests that you consult with a gynecologist.

Dear Impotents Anonymous:

My husband is sixty-three. A hernia operation rendered him impotent about ten years ago. Testosterone helped. Then about five years ago cancer of the prostate, subsequent surgery, and radiation therapy completed the process. So he had a penile implant.

At first we had sex once or twice a week. But for the last two years, he hasn't expressed any interest in it.

About a year ago he started accusing me of going with other men. He avoids the psychiatrist and is suspicious of him. At times he has become violent. Can you recommend a therapist who might be experienced with this type of difficulty? We have been married for thirty-five years and I don't want to leave him, but he frightened me so that I did leave about a week ago. We need help desperately.

A. A.
Sioux Falls, SD

Dear A. A.:

Thank you for writing, and I hope that your circumstances are changing for the better. I would highly suggest that you seek psychological or marriage counseling, even if your husband refuses to go. There is more going on with your relationship than impotence. And you need to take positive action as soon as possible.

If you would like a referral, please call me at Impotents Anonymous headquarters.

WE CAN'T AFFORD TREATMENT

Dear Impotents Anonymous:

We enjoyed your videocassette and we understand that we need help. Our problem is that we lack money for treatment. I am in my seventies and on Social Security. My wife, who also is retired, wants normal sex. How can we get help?

R. S.
Manchester, NH

Dear R. S.:

First of all, you should consult with a urologist specialist to determine the cause of your impotence. Medicare will cover part of the cost for the testing and diagnosis. You can ask your doctor for specific details.

The cost of external management devices, should your urologist recommend one, is very reasonable: $200 to $300. Many people are very satisfied with them.

Dear Impotents Anonymous:

I am fifty-two years old and have had an erection problem for two years. I took testosterone last year and it helped a little; but it was very expensive. I had to stop it due to side effects.

My doctor told me that a penile implant would put me out of work for three months. I cannot afford that. Do you have any alternatives for helping with erection problems?

R. L.
Syracuse, NY

Dear R. L.:

Today there are a number of alternatives available besides penile implants: penile injection therapy (PEP) and external management devices. In addition, some penile implant surgeries can be done on an outpatient basis, saving even more money. You should discuss these options with your urologist.

Our National Medical Advisor tells us that you should not miss more than two to three weeks of work after receiving a penile implant. Some doctors recommend six weeks if you do heavy lifting.

Dear Impotents Anonymous:

I received a copy of your newsletter from a friend and I am enclosing a check for a subscription.

I would like to receive a list of the meetings around my area, which is Georgia, Florida, and Alabama. I am in a wheelchair and I receive SSI. Does Medicaid pay for the operation? Could you tell me if any financial bureau will help, or if you have a payment plan for a penile prosthesis? Any help you could give me would be greatly appreciated. Thank you.

S. M.
Mobile, AL

Dear S. M.:

Thank you so much for your letter and for your subscription to our newsletter.

Enclosed is a meeting list that covers the states you mentioned. I hope you can find a chapter location convenient to you.

At this time I do not think that Medicaid pays for the operation, but I do believe Medicare does, at least a great part of it. Your best approach is to consult with a urologist who could have a far better idea of what financial help is available in your particular area.

We do not sell the prosthesis. I do know of several members of I.A., both paraplegic and quadriplegic, who have had the surgery. And they are very pleased with the results.

Dear Bruce and Eileen:

I would like to express my great appreciation to the I.A. and I-Anon organizations and to Eileen and Bruce, its founders, for the support and encouragement they have given me.

As you know, I had lots of explanations, but no support, from doctors when they found out my insurance carrier would not pay the medical expenses for a penile implant. It was only because your National Medical Advisor, Dr. Myron Murdock, took enough interest in my case to challenge the insurance company that they reversed their decision and paid all medical costs.

I am very happy with the results. And I can never thank you and Dr. Murdock enough.

L. S.
Arlington, VA

STOP PLAYING DOCTOR

Dear Impotents Anonymous:

I am seventy-four years old. I have had gradual impotence coming on. When I put a rubber band around the base of my penis, it helps. But it is not good enough. Can you make any suggestions?

T. W.
Chattanooga, TN

Dear T. W.:

Do not, *under any circumstances,* use a rubber band to trap blood in your penis. Doing so could cause serious injury.

First, you should consult with a urologist specialist to find out what is causing your impotence problem. Impotence can be a symptom of an underlying medical problem that may even be life-threatening. Ignoring this warning signal and attempting to treat yourself on your own is asking for trouble.

If your urologist believes an external management device will help you overcome the effects of your impotence, there are relatively inexpensive FDA-approved devices that are safe to use.

Dear Bruce and Eileen:

I received the enclosed letter and pamphlet from you about fifteen months ago.

I went to one of the doctors you suggested in San Francisco. He gave me an examination and said my hormone level was borderline so he gave me testosterone. It helped some, but I had to take about four capsules a day and that went on for three months. My feet blew up but I could tell it helped some. But I still could not have complete intercourse.

I get erections at night good enough to have sex. But when I start, it will not hold up long enough. I cannot get erections in the daytime and I don't have any feeling for sex, only in the morning before I get up.

Frequently I get mail trying to sell me some pills. But I don't trust them. I do trust you for I believe you are honest.

H. S.
Butte, MT

Dear H. S.:

I'm glad to know that you did receive a certain amount of help through testosterone treatments. However, based on what you say, it appears that it is not the total answer.

You should know that there are now injection treatments which many doctors are using at this time. There are also external management devices that have been FDA approved. You should discuss all of this with your doctor.

Concerning the pills advertised in the magazines, we do not have details. But before using any, consult with your doctor. We do not express any opinions concerning products manufactured by nonmembers of the institutes.

Please keep in touch about your progress.

Dear Impotents Anonymous:

The magazine *50 Plus* has suggested that I write your agency for information on impotence.

I am seventy-one years old and have had two TURs [prostate surgery]. I am otherwise in good health and have married again after thirteen years of sexual inactivity.

My problem now is three years of lack of ejaculation. Have you any literature on this condition?

T. N.
Cardston, Alberta, Canada

Dear T. N.:

Impotence is the inability to gain and maintain an erection long enough to successfully complete intercourse. From the description in your letter, I cannot be certain that this is your problem. It's obvious, though, that you are concerned about this situation.

Stop playing doctor and consult with your urologist about your problem. Only after a complete evaluation will he be able to tell you what to do to overcome your difficulties. If you want a referral to a specialist in your area, please call our headquarters.

Dear I-Anon:

To whom it may concern: I've been married to my sweetheart for two and a half months. I've known him for nine years. Every time we make love, he becomes impotent. What could cause that? He used to brag about his bachelor days in the navy, and now that we married, it's like he can't. He's only twenty-nine years old. This has been going on for over a year. Could it be me and he's not telling me?

Y. P.
Provo, UT

Dear Y. P.:

Thank you for your letter.

Since nearly 75 percent of impotence is caused by a physical problem, the odds suggest that the problem is with him and not with you. However, you cannot be certain about what is causing his impotence until he goes to a urologist specialist for a complete evaluation.

I encourage you to seek help as soon as possible. Impotence may be the symptom of a serious, sometimes life-threatening medical problem. You should not put off his seeing a urologist.

Dear Mr. and Mrs. MacKenzie:

Please send me whatever information you can to relieve my inability to achieve an erection.

This affliction has come on in the past fifteen years. It began gradually. It coincided almost exactly with my use of high blood pressure medication. But I failed to recognize the connection.

I no longer take this medication. (I no longer eat salty foods—pretzels, sauerkraut, olives, potato chips, peanuts, etc.) But my problem persists.

I am now fifty-seven years old. Needless to say I used to be virile—perhaps unusually virile. I have four children.

A. N.
Lynchburg, VA

Dear A. N.:

The high blood pressure medication that you mentioned certainly could have contributed to the onset of your impotence. Now that you are no longer on the medication, though, you should be seeing an improvement in your condition—unless there is another medical problem going on.

Impotence may be a symptom of a potentially life-threatening disease process. You should not ignore this symptom. You should see a urologist specialist as soon as possible.

Dear Impotents Anonymous:

I am enclosing a self-addressed envelope. Please forward your booklet "Answers to the Most Asked Questions About Chronic Impotence."

May I ask a personal question? What can a seventy-eight-year-old man, who rarely can achieve an erection and who is living with a woman who enjoys sex and can achieve orgasm, do?

Surely this is an age-old question. I am not asking for the Fountain of Youth, but in this day of mechanical and electronic ingenuity, what can be done?

V. B.
Fairbanks, AK

Dear V. B.:

Yes, it is an age-old question—and you are not expecting the Fountain of Youth, just a normal, warm sexual relationship with a partner you care for.

Yes, today there are many options available for helping you overcome the effects of your impotence. First, however, you need to seek an accurate diagnosis of your condition from a urologist specialist. Impotence may be the symptom of a serious, even life-threatening, disease process. You should not delay finding out what is causing your problem.

Dear Impotents Anonymous:

I am thirty-seven years old and have recently experienced a problem with impotence. I have seen my family doctor and a local urologist who have examined me and performed some blood-chemistry testing. These examinations and test results show no apparent cause for the problem, and my doctors have no suggestions or recommendations for treatment.

The problem continues and I would like to contact a physician who may be more knowledgeable and experienced in the treatment of impotence. I see a number of devices and pills advertised in magazines I get. Do you think they would work? I'm ready to try anything.

K. N.
Tempe, AZ

Dear K. N.:

I'm afraid your story is all too common. Many family physicians and even urologists do not know how to correctly diagnose and treat chronic impotence. Only one in three urologists specializes in impotence. If you would like a referral to a specialist, you can call our headquarters.

We do not comment regarding the pills and unapproved devices advertised in magazines. You should consult with a urologist specialist before trying them.

You should know that today there are many options for treating and for overcoming the effects of chronic impotence. No man need remain impotent.

Dear Impotents Anonymous:

Due to my impotence problem, I am interested in locating a good urologist in my area. I am in the Providence, RI, area. I have seen my family physician and he laughs at the situation and suggests "keep trying," his only remark!

Due to this fact, I'd like a second opinion. I'm sixty-six and in good physical health, and feel I have a good life ahead.

Thank you kindly for any assistance.

R. B.
Cranston, RI

Dear R. B.:

It's unfortunate that many family physicians are not informed about impotence. A decade ago most doctors thought that 90 percent of impotence was caused by emotional problems. Today, however, we believe that at least 65 to 75 percent of impotence is related to a physical problem.

I suggest that you consult with one of the urologists in your area who specializes in the diagnosis and treatment of impotence. I've enclosed the names of three. You do have a good life ahead of you, and you should not give up until you get your answer.

Dear Impotents Anonymous:

I saw your program on impotence on the "20/20" show. I have done some research on this subject and found out that alcohol, spicy food, citrus food and juices, and apples and apple juice are foods to stay away from when you are having a problem with impotence.

I started taking vitamins B, B_2, E, and zinc. This helps some.

Please send me any information you have. I am a male forty-eight years old in good physical shape. I work out three times a week and I'm six feet tall and weigh 160 pounds.

L. A.
Orlando, FL

Dear L. A.:

Unless you have a diagnosed vitamin deficiency, our National Medical Advisor says that it is unlikely that vitamins will help your impotence.

I'm not certain where you got the information on the specific foods you mentioned, but we do not have any documented research supporting this recommendation. We do know, however, that alcohol, and nicotine from smoking, can adversely affect potency.

Rather than trying to become a self-taught expert, I suggest that you consult with a urologist specialist who can accurately diagnose the cause of your problem. Only then will you be able to select a treatment plan that will help restore your potency or help you overcome the effects of your impotence.

Dear Impotents Anonymous:

I read in the *Intisari Magazin* the article titled "Impotensi Anonymous." I would like to get some information from you about the new medicine that can cure my problem. I have a problem having an erection and I cannot do my task as a husband.

Would you be so kind as to give me information about that medicine. Where can I buy it? Can we find it in hospitals in Indonesia or in the drugstore?

I am waiting for your information. Thank you for your help.

K. C.
Indonesia

Dear K. C.:

Thank you for your inquiry. It is important for you to know that appropriate medical testing and evaluation should be done to ascertain whether the cause of your impotence is physical or psychological.

You should consult with a urologist who has expertise in dealing with erectile dysfunction. We shall institute inquiries among our associate members and professional members for the names of physicians in Indonesia who may be of help to you. When I have those names, I shall be pleased to send them to you. You should know that there is help available for all men suffering with this problem.

Dear Impotents Anonymous:

Can you be of any assistance? For some years I've had a problem of relative impotence—partial erections only. Occasional nightly erections. My desire is still strong.

I am taking a blood pressure pill. My general health is excellent. I eat and sleep well and have an attractive wife. Generally, I feel as though I were in my forties.

Can you be of any assistance? Changes in diet? Medicines? Temporarily discontinue blood pressure pills?

G. S.
Albany, GA

Dear G. S.:

Do not stop taking your blood pressure medication without first checking with your physician. Doing so could be very dangerous. Blood pressure medication has been associated with impotence, and perhaps your doctor can recommend a different type, or dosage, and relieve your problem.

To our knowledge, there is no evidence that diet has any effect on impotence.

Impotence may be the symptom of a serious, sometimes life-threatening medical problem. Therefore, I suggest that you consult with a urologist specialist as soon as possible to determine the cause of your impotence. Only then will you know the options available to you for overcoming your problem.

Dear Impotents Anonymous:

I am a healthy male and I've never had venereal diseases. I had a circumcision when I was forty and a vasectomy eight years later (before my present marriage). We had adequate sexual relations the first year or two.

About two years ago my ability to have erections disappeared. We've had no sexual relations the last three years. We are both very religious and believe in fidelity and marital chastity. I even feel guilty when lustful ideas cross my mind!

I am starting a regimen of supplementing my diet with natural vitamins C, A, B, and D. I also started taking zinc. Also I am trying to "psych" myself into a proper attitude to regain my potency.

Any information you can give me which will help me to recover my ability to have erections would be appreciated.

H. A.
Ely, NV

Dear H. A.:

According to our National Medical Advisor, unless you have a diagnosed vitamin deficiency, there is no study that demonstrates that taking vitamins will help restore your potency.

You are trying to play doctor, as Bruce and I did. Trying to "psych" yourself into a proper attitude is ignoring the fact that 75 percent of impotence is caused by a physical problem requiring medical attention.

I strongly suggest that you consult with a urologist specialist in your area to find out the cause of your impotence. Then you will be able to select a proper course of action for overcoming your problem.

Dear I-Anon:

I buy *Woman's Day* magazine once a month. In the last issue, I saw the article titled "Marriage: A Husband's Impotence; A Wife's Dilemma." One part says "unable to get or maintain an erection sufficient for intercourse," which is my husband's trouble now. At the end of the article I saw your recommendation about a [sex] therapy, which I feel I need now. Can you help me find a sex therapist certified by AASECT (American Association of Sex Educators, Counselors and Therapists)? Thank you very much.

G. M.
Lowell, MA

Dear G. M.:

Thank you for your letter. Before giving any referrals, I should like to point out one or two facts. Nearly 75 percent of impotence is due to physical causes. Therefore, before consulting with a sex therapist, your husband should see a urologist specialist to determine the cause of his problem. Should the problem be psychogenic, then sex therapy may be in order.

Many marital relationships deteriorate because of the stress caused by impotence. Even if your husband has a physical problem, you and he may need some marital counseling or sex therapy to help you improve your relationship. If he refuses to go, you may wish to seek counseling for yourself. No reputable sex therapist will treat your husband's impotence without first requesting a complete evaluation from a urologist.

I've enclosed the names of several urologist specialists and psychologists in your area who specialize in the treatment of impotence.

Dear Impotents Anonymous:

I know somebody from your group can help me with my problem. I am forty-six and have low blood pressure.

My problem is my inability to achieve a satisfactory erection or, when I do, it dies down in the middle of my partner's excitement. This condition always leads to a violent quarrel with my girlfriend of three years—accusing me of such things as I don't like her anymore, or maybe I have a new girlfriend.

What vitamins would you suggest for an improved erection? I read about a test for male impotence that measures the force of an erection during sleep. But in my case, the only time I get an erection during sleep is when I feel like urinating. How reliable is this test? Am I qualified for your group?

J. W.
Saudi Arabia

Dear J. W.:

Vitamins are not normally suggested to help a person with erection problems. The tests for male impotence that measure erections during sleep are the nocturnal penile tumescence (NPT) test, the Dacomed Snap Gauge test, or the Rigiscan. In addition, a solution of papaverine and Regitine injected directly into the base of the penis can demonstrate if you are physically capable of having an erection. All of these tests should be supervised and the results interpreted by a urologist specialist.

Are you taking medicine for your low blood pressure problem? Medications for blood pressure problems very often cause impotence. You should check this out with a urologist. Perhaps your medication should be changed.

We shall be very glad to hear from you again. If you wish a referral, we shall do our best to give you one. There is help available for your problem.

GLOSSARY

angiogram/angiography: A diagnostic X ray used to locate specific blood-vessel blockage and thus indicate if a penile blood-flow problem can be corrected surgically.

aphrodisiac: A substance thought to increase sexual desire (libido) and improve sexual performance. See also *yohimbine.*

bypass: An operative procedure that reroutes blood to avoid obstruction in vessels.

catheter: A rubber or plastic tube inserted through the urethra to the bladder to permit urine to exit from bladder.

cavernosagram: A diagnostic X ray used to locate (dye is injected) venous leakage from the penis.

corpora cavernosa: Two spongy rodlike structures above the urethra in the penis that trap blood for the erection.

corpus spongiosum: A rodlike structure located in the middle and beneath the urethra (urinary tube) of the penis that also becomes erect.

cystometrogram: A diagnostic test used to detect if the penis is receiving "messages" through the nerves from the brain.

electrostimulatory device: See *Male Electronic Genital Stimulator.*

endarterectomy: A surgical procedure used to remove plaque (blockage) and damaged tissue from an artery to improve blood flow to the penis.

endocrinologist: A physician specializing in hormones.

engorgement: The filling (beyond tumescence) of the penis with blood during an erection to the point of achieving rigidity.

entrapment device: An external management device used to trap blood in the penis so the man can achieve an erection.

erection: An increased volume of blood flowing to the penis that causes the penis to become enlarged (tumescent) and rigid (engorged).

estrogen: The female sex hormone that is associated with supporting female secondary sexual characteristics, such as enlarged breasts, rounded hips, pubic hair, and so forth. See also *testosterone.*

excising: Surgical removal of, for example, plaque.

external management device: A device that is applied to the outside of the penis and that enables a man to gain and maintain an erection to complete intercourse; for example, an entrapment or vacuum device.

fibrosis: Scar tissue.

flaccidity: The limp state the penis assumes when not erect.

follicle-stimulating hormone (FSH): Stimulates the cells of the testicles that produce sperm.

fully inflatable penile implant: A surgically implanted (totally concealed) penile prosthesis that includes a fluid reservoir, two inflatable penile cylinders, and a pump with a deflate mechanism.

glans penis: The tip or head of the penis; part of the corpus spongiosum.

hinged penile implant: A surgically implanted (totally concealed) penile prosthesis that has a hingelike action at the base of the penis so it can be placed in an upright or flaccid position.

hypothalamus: The portion of the brain located on the under surface near the pituitary gland, and which affects its function.

impotence: The inability to gain and maintain an erection through the completion of successful intercourse.

impotence, chronic: The persistence of impotence for five or more weeks.

impotence, physical: Impotence caused by an organic problem such as vascular disease, neuropathy, reaction to medications or toxic substances, and so forth. Accounts for nearly 75 percent of chronic impotence.

impotence, primary: Impotence that has persisted since birth; characterized by never having achieved an erection.

impotence, psychogenic: Impotence caused by an emotional problem such as depression, performance anxiety, or stress. Accounts for about 25 percent of chronic impotence.

impotence, secondary: Impotence having an onset sometime after birth due to the development of a physical or psychological problem, or a combination of both.

impotence, temporary: Usually a sudden onset of impotence associated with illness, the death of a spouse, or after another life crisis. It often resolves itself or responds to counseling.

impotence, vasculogenic: Impotence caused as a result of reduced blood flow due to contraction of arteries.

impotence, venogenic: Impotence caused by the failure of the venous valves (polsters) to trap blood in the penis.

incising: Surgical cutting of, for example, plaque.

incontinence: The inability to control urination.

internal erection device: See *penile implant.*

libido: Sexual desire.

luteinizing hormone (LH): Stimulates the cells of the testicles that produce testosterone.

Male Electronic Genital Stimulator (MEGS): A self-contained, battery-operated device that can be inserted into the anus to stimulate, through a mild electric current, an erection.

malleable penile implant: A surgically implanted (totally concealed) prosthesis that has two flexible cores which "remember" the position they are placed in.

Mercury String Gauge: "Wires" used in sleep testing.

MMPI (Minnesota Multiphase Personality Inventory): A psychological evaluation test.

neuropathy: Nerve damage often associated with diabetes.

NPT (nocturnal penile tumescence) test: An evaluation indicating quality, quantity, and duration of girth in the penis.

papaverine: A drug used to dilate blood vessels.

penile implant: A surgically implanted (totally concealed) prosthesis inserted into the penis; includes semirigid, hinged, malleable, self-contained (fluid, segmented), and fully inflatable types.

performance anxiety: The fear of failure.

Peyronie's disease: The deposition of scar tissue in the shaft of the penis, probably due to the inflammation of blood vessels in the penis.

pharmacological erection program (PEP): A nonsurgical approach to the treatment of impotence; a penile injection of, for example, papaverine/Regitine.

phentolamine mesylate: A drug used to dilate arteries and constrict veins.

polsters: Valves in the veins through which blood leaves the penis. See *impotence, venogenic.*

priapism: An unwanted, sustained, and painful erection that, if left untreated, may damage the valves in the veins leaving the penis as well as other delicate penile structures.

prolactin: A hormone commonly associated with nursing (lactating) mothers; an excess of this hormone causes decreased testosterone production, which may lead to impotence. See also *testosterone.*

prolonged erection: A priapismlike erection that can be a side effect of the PEP self-injection program; requires immediate medical intervention to avoid damage to delicate penile structures.

prostaglandin: A hormone that, when injected into the penis, can cause an erection. See also *pharmacological erection program* (*PEP*).

pudendal nerve: A main nerve to the penis, which has a sensory and movement function.

pudendal nerve conduction time: A diagnostic test that determines whether or not the pudendal nerve serving the penis is intact.

radio immunoassay (RIA) blood test: Biological test in which radioactive antigen antibody complexes are used to determine quantitative levels of testosterone.

radionucleotide penogram: A relatively new penile blood-flow test used to "picture" the blood flowing through the vessels in the penis.

refractory period: Following ejaculation, the physical recovery period required before another erection can be achieved.

Regitine: See *phentolamine mesylate.*

retrograde ejaculation: When ejaculate discharges into bladder rather than through the urethra.

revascularization: Utilizing a blood vessel from another part of the body to replace an inadequate vessel.

rigidity: The engorgement of the penis with blood to the point that the penis becomes stiff. See also *engorgement.*

Rigiscan: A diagnostic instrument used to test the quality, quantity, and duration of nighttime erections.

semirigid penile implant: Two totally concealed, semirigid, flexible plastic rods surgically inserted into the penis.

sensate focus exercises: Therapeutic exercises to improve sexual function by making individuals more aware of the sensual aspects of their bodies.

Snap Gauge: A home-performed sleep test used to detect the presence of nighttime erections.

steal syndrome: The loss of an erection when the effort of intercourse (in some positions) causes lower extremities to "steal" the blood supply from the penis.

testicle: Found as a pair in the scrotum (male pouch or sac behind penis), these round medium-soft male components play a major role in the manufacture of testosterone.

testosterone: The male hormone responsible for sexual desire (libido) and for secondary sexual characteristics, such as a deep voice, pubic hair, and so forth.

transurethral resection: Removal of the center portion of an enlarged and obstructed prostate gland using a procedure whereby the cutting instruments enter through the urethral opening.

tumescence: Enlargement (girth) of the penis caused by increased blood flow. See also *engorgement.*

urologist: A physician who treats the male genitourinary tract. Only about one in three urologists specializes in diagnosing and treating impotence.

vacuum erection device: An external management device that pulls a gentle vacuum on the penis and causes it to engorge with blood.

vasoactive intestinal peptide (VIP): A group of amino acids that trigger nerve transmitters at nerve endings, thereby increasing blood flow.

vasoconstrictor: Drug that causes blood vessels to decrease in diameter.

vasodilator: a medication that can improve penile blood flow by expanding the blood vessels.

yohimbine: An aphrodisiac that can improve the performance of the nerves serving the penis.

INDEX